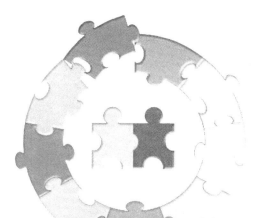

Care Coordination and **Transition**

Management (CCTM)

REVIEW QUESTIONS

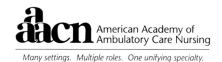
American Academy of
Ambulatory Care Nursing

Many settings. Multiple roles. One unifying specialty.

© Copyright 2016
American Academy of Ambulatory Care Nursing
East Holly Avenue Box 56, Pitman, NJ 08071-0056
Phone: 856-256-2350 or 800-AMB-NURS; Fax: 856-589-7463
e-mail: aaacn@ajj.com; website: www.aaacn.com

ISBN: 978-1-940325-27-9

All rights reserved. No part of this publication, except the answer sheets, may be reproduced, distributed, or transmitted in any form or by any means, electronic or mechanical, including but not limited to, the process of scanning and digitization, photocopying, recording, or any information storage and retrieval systems without the written permission of the American Academy of Ambulatory Care Nursing.

Suggested Citation
Leaver, C.A. (Ed.). *Care coordination and transition management review questions.*
Pitman, NJ: American Academy of Ambulatory Care Nursing.

Publication Management by
Anthony J. Jannetti, Inc.
East Holly Avenue Box 56
Pitman, NJ 08071-0056
www.ajj.com

CCTM Review Questions Task Force Contributors

Chair of CCTM Review Question Task Force, Editor, and Contributor

Cynthia A. Leaver, PhD, APRN, FNP-BC
Associate Dean of Faculty and Research
United States University, College of Nursing
San Diego, CA

Senior Advisor and Contributor

Candia Baker Laughlin, MS, RN-BC
Past President, AAACN
Ann Arbor, MI

Board Liaison and Contributor

Rocquel Crawley, DHA, MBA, BSN, RNC-OB, NEA-BC
Director of Nursing and Operations, Ambulatory Care
VCU Health System
Richmond, VA

Contributors

Mary "Molly" Benkert, MS, RN-BC, CBIS
Nurse Program Manager/Nurse Care Coordinator
Denver Health/Denver HCP for Children and Your with
Special Health Care Needs
Denver, CO

Sarah L. Flores, MS, RN-BC,
Manager, Specialty Clinics
CHOC Children's Hospital
Orange, CA

Mary Anne Granger, MSN, RN
Clinical Resource Leader Care Coordination
Ambulatory Care Services
Maricopa Integrated Health Services
Phoenix, AZ

Christine M. Griffel, MSN, RN-BC
Registered Nurse Care Manager
Veterans Administration Pittsburgh Healthcare System
Pittsburgh, PA

Pamella Guntrum, DNP, MSN, RN-C
Ambulatory & Allied Care Services
Manager, Clinical Development & Patient Education
UW Medicine-Harborview Medical Center
Seattle, WA

Dwight Hampton, MBA, BSN, RN-BC, PCMH, CCE
Deputy Director, Diversity and Inclusion
Navy Bureau of Medicine and Surgery
Falls Church, VA

Edtrina Moss, PhD(c), MSN, RN-BC, NE-BC
Utilization Review/Utilization Management RN
Veterans Health Administration
Houston, TX

Lois Stauffer, MSN, RN, CNL
Manager, Care Coordination
OhioHealth Physician Group
Dublin, OH

Tamara Templeton, BSN, RN-BC
PACT Care Coordinator
Veterans Health Administration
Gainesville, FL

David Thomas, MPA, BSN, CEN, CMSRN, RN-BC, PLNC
Deputy Director for Medical Services, Navy Ambulatory
Care Nursing Specialty Leader
Naval Hospital Bremerton, WA
Bremerton, WA

Introduction

Welcome to the *Care Coordination and Transition Management (CCTM) Review Questions* published by the American Academy of Ambulatory Care Nursing (AAACN). This set of mock test items is designed to assist nurses in assessing their knowledge of the practice of care coordination and transition management, and to prepare for the Certified in Care Coordination and Transition Management (CCCTM) exam provided by the Medical-Surgical Nursing Certification Board (MSNCB) in collaboration with AAACN. Professional nurses should take every opportunity to advance their expertise, skills, and knowledge, and use tools such as this publication to assess their knowledge gaps and learn from studying the answers.

All the review questions, and their answers, associated page numbers, and rationales (found in the back of the book) are based on the *Care Coordination and Transition Management Core Curriculum* (Haas, Swan, & Haynes, 2014), an AAACN publication. Using this *Core Curriculum* as the companion to this set of review questions is highly recommended. For more information on care coordination and transition management (CCTM), access: https://www.aaacn.org/cctm

The *CCTM Review Questions* reflect the latest test blueprint of the CCTM exam. The multiple-choice items are grouped into *six* domains of practice, with the percentage of questions for each domain based upon the CCCTM exam blueprint (see Table 1). The content in each of the domains is drawn from the *CCTM Core Curriculum.*

Table 1.

Category	Domain of Practice	Percentage	Number of Review Questions
I	Communication and transition throughout the care continuum	20%	40
II	Education, engagement, coaching, and counseling of patients, caregivers, and support network	20%	40
III	Population health management	20%	40
IV	Patient-centered care planning and support for self-management	15%	30
V	Teamwork and interprofessional collaboration	15%	30
VI	Advocacy	10%	20

Exam Information

The Certified in Care Coordination and Transition Management (CCCTM) exam was developed by nurses practicing care coordination and transition management under the expert guidance of the Center for Nursing Education and Testing (C-NET). It is a computer-based exam containing 150 multiple-choice questions. A standard score of 95 (approximately 72%) is required to pass. Candidates have 3 hours to take the exam.

Complete information about the exam, exam blueprint, application, and testing process is available on MSNCB's website http://www.msncb.org/cctm, msncb@msncb.org, or 866-877-2676. AAACN offers a variety of CCCTM exam study resources. For more information, visit https://www.aaacn.org/cctm. The exam is offered at C-NET testing sites across the country. To locate a testing site near you and find further information about testing, access: http://www.cnetnurse.com/test-site-locations/computer-based-locations/ The CCCTM certification is valid for 5 years. The two options to recertify are by continuing education or taking the exam.

Recommendations for Using These Review Questions

1. Complete all multiple-choice items or focus upon the items specific to one or more of the above domains.
2. Read each multiple-choice item carefully and circle your answer on the Answer Sheets provided at the end of this publication.
   - Try to answer the question before reading the options.
   - Underline key words.
   - Do not read anything more into the question or options than what is there; do not over analyze.
   - If unsure of the answer, use logic to rule out options that could be correct versus those that are definitely incorrect.
   - Select options that reflect a nursing judgment.
   - If two answers are correct, choose the one that causes the other to occur.
   - Select the option that is correct without exception.
   - In the evaluation of difficult test questions, mark out the options you think are wrong.
   - Avoid options that are true statements but do not answer the question.

3. Check for the correct answers using the Answer Key located at the end of this publication. For further information about the topic addressed in the question and the rationale for the answer given, reference the *CCTM Core Curriculum*, and the page listed.
4. There is no passing score for this assessment. Reward yourself for the items you answer correctly. Review those items that you answer incorrectly to determine your areas for further study.

Disclaimer: These review questions provide an opportunity to assess CCTM nursing practice and to prepare for answering multiple-choice items. They do not represent a comprehensive compilation of all content composing CCTM nursing practice. Completion of these review questions does not guarantee the examinee will pass the CCCTM exam. The editor and reviewers of these review questions are *not* CCCTM Test Development Committee members or item writers.

The names used in the case examples in this publication are fictitious and not based on any real or actual patient or nurse.

Reference

Haas, S.A., Swan, B.A., & Haynes, T.S. (2014). *Care coordination and transition management core curriculum*. Pitman, NJ: American Academy of Ambulatory Care Nursing.

Questions 1-3 refer to the following patient case.

Melisa Kelly, a 57-year-old patient hospitalized with pneumonia, is being discharged to home. The nurse care coordinator has identified Ms. Kelly as high risk for readmission and sent a message to her primary care provider's nurse care coordinator.

1. What **CRITICAL** information should be included in the communication from the acute care case manager?
   A. Chart summary, medication reconciliation, and discharge instructions.
   B. Follow-up appointments and pharmacies the patient has used in the last year.
   C. Discharge instructions, functional status for independent activities of daily living, and transportation mode at discharge.
   D. Allergy list, problem list, and description of medication adherence for the past 12 months.

2. Following discharge, the nurse care coordinator contacts Ms. Kelly at home. Ms. Kelly states, "They gave me a list of medications I'm supposed to be taking, but I don't have all of them here at home." What should the nurse care coordinator do next?
   A. Make an appointment with Ms. Kelly's primary care provider in the next week and reassure her to just take the medications she has until she sees her provider.
   B. Instruct Ms. Kelly to contact her pharmacies used in the last 12 months to see if they might have prescriptions on hand for those medications.
   C. Validate the name, dose, route, and frequency of all medications on the discharge medication list and compare with what Ms. Kelly has at home.
   D. Call the hospitalist and clarify if any of these medications should be discontinued, and request prescriptions for those that are missing.

3. The nurse care coordinator is looking for the social worker's notes from Ms. Kelly's inpatient stay. The nurse care coordinator cannot find them in the medical record and calls the unit from which Ms. Kelly was discharged. The nurse care coordinator is told social workers do not document on the same platform as the rest of the inpatient documentation. What can health systems do to prevent this type of barrier?
   A. Promote use of order sets, alerts, and standard plans of care to aid in error prevention.
   B. Promote access for all care team members to a common documentation platform.
   C. Advocate for use of smart sets and standardized templates for social workers for planning discharges, and advocate for imaging of social work notes into the archived record.
   D. Acquire handheld documentation hardware and software for social workers and develop standardized training for them.

4. A patient is hospitalized for knee replacement surgery. She will be discharged home today with home health nurse and physical therapy visits. The nurse care coordinator notices the patient has a history of mild congestive heart failure and Type 2 diabetes. What should the nurse care coordinator **PRIMARILY** consider when planning communications for transitional care for this patient?
   A. The patient is not at significant risk for readmission, so the nurse care coordinator should assure the surgeon's office has information needed for follow-up.
   B. Since the home health professionals will see the patient, the patient will not need to be contacted by the nurse care coordinator after discharge.
   C. The nurse care coordinator should collect all pertinent data regarding the patient's discharge plan of care and follow-up with the patient's family.
   D. Communication gaps between providers in acute care, specialists, home care, and primary care may create incomplete or fragmented information that the care coordinator will need to address.

5. Which of the following models enhance communication and collaboration between acute care and ambulatory care providers during transitions of care?
   A. Patient Activation Measure® (PAM®).
   B. Patients at Risk for Rehospitalization (PARR).
   C. Better Outcomes by Optimizing Transitions (BOOST) tool – 8Ps.
   D. Centers for Medicare & Medicaid Quality Review and Utilization (QRUR).

6. How would one most accurately describe the characteristics of a high-quality transition of care?
   A. Patients' needs identified by specialty providers are addressed only by that specialty in the ambulatory setting.
   B. Communication practices of care providers minimize risks associated with handoffs across transitions of care, such as through using SBAR or I-PASS.
   C. Events at transition of care are reflected in the medical record for accurate billing and coding.
   D. The patient or member of the patient's family is assigned a team leader role for care transitions and is provided with focused instructions.

7. In what manner do information systems and technology assist in preventing error and support safe care transitions?
   A. Information systems can contain alerts and practice advisories to aid in care transitions.
   B. Interoperability between information systems and knowledge management systems guarantees patient understanding of the plan of care even with multiple provider instructions.
   C. Patients can elect to have personal health information sent to their personal email address for sharing with health care providers in the future.
   D. Information system security and access are the only way to prevent Health Insurance Portability and Accountability Act (HIPAA) violations at care transitions.

Questions 8 and 9 refer to the following patient case.

Jenny Williams is a 47-year-old with Stage 4 breast cancer. She is being discharged following surgery for removal of metastatic lung tumors.

8. Which answer **BEST** describes patient-centered care in planning for Ms. Williams' transition from acute care?
   A. Goals for care created by the inpatient case manager are useful only in the inpatient setting, and the ambulatory care team needs to begin a new assessment of the patient's and family's needs and goals.
   B. End-of-life ethical and legal issues should be referred to the patient's spiritual and legal advisor to resolve with the patient.
   C. Involvement in decision-making is deferred until Ms. Williams has regained her strength and is not taking narcotic pain medication.
   D. Patient and caregiver concerns are identified and integrated into a plan of care which engages Ms. Williams and her family in setting goals and managing symptoms as the disease progresses.

9. The inpatient case manager has identified gaps in Ms. Williams' health literacy and problems with transportation to her follow-up appointments. What actions can the community-based nurse care coordinator take for Ms. Williams, after she is discharged, to help close these gaps?
   A. Send educational materials to Ms. Williams' home to have her review before her next office visit.
   B. Advise Ms. Williams too many missed appointments may cause her primary care provider to discharge her from the practice.
   C. Send Ms. Williams a questionnaire to assess her psychosocial needs.
   D. Link Ms. Williams to community resources for additional support for transportation.

10. Which of the following is considered an example of a transition of care that would benefit from the involvement of a nurse care coordinator?
    A. Transfer of patient from one room to another within the same hospital unit.
    B. Transfer of patient from pediatric primary care to adult primary care at age 18.
    C. Change-of-shift in the hospital transferring from one nurse to another.
    D. Development of patient care plan by a home care nurse for assignment to a home health aide.

11. Effective communication at transitions of care has which of the following characteristics?
    A. Mutual respect and shared decision-making within nursing and interprofessional teams.
    B. A common communication method is supported by health care informatics within the hospital.
    C. Episodic patient information obtained through phone calls and texts is conveyed through emails and hard copy notes.
    D. Documentation supports a complete problem list and proper coding for insurance plans and pharmacy benefits.

12. How can a nurse care coordinator demonstrate valuing the diversity of the patient?
    A. Respond to the patient with a standardized plan of care addressing a broad disease-based problem.
    B. Engage an interpreter when it is evident the patient is from another cultural group whose primary language is not English.
    C. Evaluate health literacy within the context of the patient's education level and life experience.
    D. Identify cultural practices the patient will need to adapt and modify in managing the disease.

13. How can a nurse care coordinator engage patients in their plan of care both during and between patient visits?
    A. Reinforce that the patient or designee is the primary source of control in his or her care.
    B. Advise patients to call their insurance case manager or community agencies if they have any questions.
    C. Refer patients to hotlines and vendor websites pertinent to their condition and its treatment.
    D. Give a provider-developed plan of care to each patient with instructions for how to follow it.

14. The **MOST** common adverse outcomes of communication failures during transitions of care are related to which of the following?
    A. Medication injuries.
    B. Falls.
    C. Readmissions.
    D. Complications related to procedures.

15. Coordination of which transition of care is **MOST** likely to positively impact health care costs?
    A. Acute care hospitalization to the primary care physician.
    B. Intensive care to general, acute inpatient care.
    C. Extended care to acute care.
    D. Primary care to specialists.

16. Which of these is a core feature or "hallmark" of transitional care?
    A. Coordination services provided for all patients being moved from a hospital setting to another care site.
    B. Differing expectations between those involved in sharing information.
    C. Focus on medically fragile patients through critical transitions in health and health care.
    D. Medication reconciliation for new medications added during the hospitalization.

17. Which of these is a risk factor for problems in cross-setting communication?
    A. Transparency and universal design of the electronic health record (EHR).
    B. Bi-directional flow of information between care teams.
    C. Failure to re-engage the primary care provider and/or team through a post-discharge office visit.
    D. Printed discharge instructions and educational materials provided to patients at discharge from the hospital.

18. What is the goal of Medicare linking hospital reimbursement to hospital readmission rates?
    A. Incentivize providers to meet many of the objectives of "Healthy People 2020."
    B. Promote high-quality health care and cost savings through reduction in after-hospital adverse events.
    C. Promote the implementation of evidence-based practices in the care of the chronically ill and medically fragile population.
    D. Incentivize cost savings by imposing reimbursement penalties for states based on readmission rates.

19. A patient is being discharged from acute care following a chronic obstructive pulmonary disease (COPD) exacerbation. The nurse care coordinator identifies the patient is unable to do a "teach-back" in the use of an inhaler. What is the **MOST** likely cause of this?
    A. The patient's insurance does not cover patient education.
    B. The patient wants to be transitioned to palliative care.
    C. The patient has poor/low health literacy.
    D. The patient has not recovered adequately and is not physically ready for discharge.

20. What did the Institute of Medicine report as the source of over 80% of health care mistakes?
    A. EHRs not being updated properly.
    B. Ineffective or absent communication.
    C. Shared information being delayed or incomplete.
    D. Lack of follow-up appointments following hospital discharge.

21. What are considered the main, foundational elements of transitional care?
    A. Mechanisms to gather and share information across care settings.
    B. Mechanisms to reconcile medication and allergy lists.
    C. Comprehensive assessments and chart summaries.
    D. Customizable EHRs.

22. Which of the following has been identified as a risk factor related to inadequate communication by the Center for Transforming Healthcare?
    A. Lack of standardized order sets between facilities.
    B. Inconsistency in health information exchange documents.
    C. Customizable EHRs with on-site order entry.
    D. Lack of standardized hand-off procedure, such as use of an SBAR tool.

23. In addition to adverse events and poor outcomes for patients, ineffective transitions of care may lead to which of the following?
    A. Avoiding procedure-related complications.
    B. Hospital readmissions within 2 weeks.
    C. Decreased costs of care.
    D. Decreased mortality and morbidity.

24. The following skills describe which of the following competencies for a nurse care coordinator: act with integrity, function competently within own scope of practice, function as a member of a health care team, and continually plan for improvement in use of self in team functioning?
    A. The ability to analyze one's own professional skill set.
    B. Team building and collaboration.
    C. Effective communication.
    D. Quality improvement.

25. A nurse care coordinator has reviewed the current research and other professional literature regarding the care of the heart failure patient population. Which of the following demonstrates the **BEST** application of this review?
    A. Modifying practice based upon clinical opinion summaries.
    B. Developing a research question and applying to the institutional review board to conduct a study.
    C. Discontinuing the continuous quality improvement program targeted to this patient population.
    D. Modifying patient education methods and tools because evidence demonstrates improved outcomes result from these changes.

26. The team leader has identified an overlap in the roles and accountabilities of the nurse care coordinator and the social worker. What would be the **MOST** effective strategy for resolving this overlap?
    A. Meet with the two team members to explore their perceptions of their roles and provide guidance.
    B. Hold daily meetings to assign duties without overlap.
    C. Provide a copy of the team policies and job descriptions for the two professionals to review.
    D. Encourage quality improvement activities to measure impact of different approaches of the two team members.

27. Which of the following describes the Bridge Model?
    A. Focuses upon the provision of palliative care through persuasion of the family when told the patient's prognosis.
    B. Provides transitional care through intensive care coordination that follows the patient from hospital through discharge and beyond.
    C. Is also called BOOST (Better Outcomes for Older Adults through Safe Transitions).
    D. Incorporates education about problem medications, such as anticoagulants and insulin.

28. At the conclusion of a patient visit, the nurse care coordinator demonstrates good communication and coordination of ongoing care by doing which of the following?
    A. Providing a printed, reconciled medication list and ensuring the next appointment is scheduled.
    B. Giving the patient a list of websites to visit for information related to his or her current problem list.
    C. Instructing the patient to call when he or she is ready for another appointment.
    D. Giving the patient a map of local emergency departments (ED) to use if he or she has any medical issues.

29. Who are the two key members of the Geriatric Resources for Assessment and Care of Elders (GRACE) team?
    A. RN and LPN.
    B. RN and physician.
    C. NP and social worker
    D. DNP and nursing scholar.

30. What is defined as "a set of actions designed to ensure the coordination and continuity of health care as patients transfer between different locations or different levels of care within the same location?"
    A. An evidence-based, coordinated transfer.
    B. Transitional care.
    C. Admission and discharge.
    D. Hand-off communication.

31. According to the American Nurses Association position statement regarding the essential role of the RN in coordination of patient care (2012), which of the following describes the nurse's role?
    A. Focus of nurse care coordination should be preventive care for the pediatric population.
    B. Advanced practice RNs are singly qualified to provide coordination of medical and nursing needs of patients.
    C. Research does not support that nurses have an important impact on patient satisfaction and care quality
    D. Patient-centered care coordination is a core professional standard and competency for all RNs.

32. Which of the following might result in a communication issue influencing transitions of care?
   A. Inadequacy of insurance coverage for home health care.
   B. Perception that care responsibility ends at discharge from the impatient setting.
   C. Advanced technology in inpatient care that cannot be reproduced in the home.
   D. Polypharmacy.

33. What program was developed by the Centers for Medicare & Medicaid Services to test transition interventions for those at high-risk for readmission following a hospitalization?
   A. Better Outcomes by Optimizing Safe Transitions (BOOST).
   B. Patient-Centered Medical Home (PCMH)
   C. Community-based Care Transitions Program (CCTP).
   D. Healthcare Effectiveness Data and Information Set (HEDIS®) measures.

34. Which elements of communication at hand-off are essential?
   A. Medication management, primary/specialty care follow-up, knowledge of red-flag warnings, and copy/access to patient-centered health record.
   B. Medication reconciliation, diagnostic reports, lab results, and detailed care plans.
   C. Family/patient education literature, medication list, allergy list, and current diagnosis.
   D. Medical records, referrals for additional care, diagnostic studies for follow-up, and directions for home care.

35. When assessing the patient to be high risk for adverse events after discharge, what might the care plan include for providing patient support and ongoing assessment?
   A. Follow-up appointment within 7 days.
   B. Complete review of systems by phone within 7 days.
   C. Contacting a cab company to take the patient home.
   D. Sending health literature to the patient in the mail.

36. A follow-up phone call within 72 hours after hospital discharge addresses what element of assessment of a patient's risk for adverse events after hospitalization?
   A. Patient support in the home.
   B. Review of all chronic illness diagnoses.
   C. Palliative care.
   D. Past medical history.

37. Poor health literacy can be addressed by which of the following actions after hospital discharge?
   A. Identifying services or benefits available based upon their diagnoses.
   B. A follow-up appointment with the primary care team.
   C. A follow-up phone call within 72 hours of discharge.
   D. Initiating a social worker referral.

38. A patient with COPD has developed severe shortness of breath. By phone, the nurse care coordinator, based upon evidence-based protocol, recommends a visit to the ED for a probable admission. How might the nurse care coordinator assist in facilitating the transfer of care to the acute setting?
   A. Notify other members of the health care team in the outpatient setting, including the primary care provider.
   B. Assure an up-to-date care medication list, including prescriptions and over-the-counter drugs and supplements, is available in the shared EHR.
   C. Ask the patient to identify his or her choice of agencies for oxygen, durable medical equipment, and home care for post-discharge planning.
   D. Coach the patient to use his or her fast-acting bronchodilator.

39. When assessing for the initiation of palliative care for a patient, which of the following interventions is most important for the care team to do **FIRST**?
   A. Discuss with the patient and family the services and benefits available.
   B. Communicate prognosis to the patient and/or family.
   C. Identify goal of care and therapeutic options.
   D. Assess and address bothersome symptoms of the patient.

40. Which answer **BEST** reflects patient engagement in self-management behaviors?
   A. Patients are advised to immediately go to the ED with any health concerns.
   B. Patients understand "sick day" insulin dosing regimens.
   C. Patients are discouraged from asking questions of their health care providers because of time constraints.
   D. Medication and treatment plan adherence is monitored by the patient's pharmacy and relayed to the provider.

Jeff Xander is a 36-year-old with cystic fibrosis (CF). He lives in a rural area, approximately 2 hours from the medical center where he receives care by a CF specialist. Mr. Xander is prescribed a 2-week course of two IV antibiotic medications to treat a pulmonary infection.

41. Which of these is the **BEST** way to establish rapport with Mr. Xander to assess his readiness for learning? Ask Mr. Xander
    A. to tell you about his previous experience with IV infusion therapy.
    B. if he prefers written instructions or written instructions with photos.
    C. to tell you all he knows about CF.
    D. about his highest level of education.

42. Mr. Xander tells you it is difficult for him to remember the sequence of the administration of his two antibiotics. Which of the following processes can support Mr. Xander's learning?
    A. Use video educational tools to provide more information and a posttest.
    B. Encourage the patient to seek training sessions on antibiotics and report lessons learned.
    C. Use pamphlets and handouts to provide more concrete information.
    D. Encourage the patient to take notes using a stable writing surface and ask questions.

43. Which of the following is an example of a question to validate Mr. Xander's understanding of medication administration? Ask Mr. Xander
    A. if he understands how to administer his medications.
    B. to state, in his own words, the sequence of the administration of his medications.
    C. about his greatest concern in administering his medications, and why this is a concern.
    D. if he feels ready to learn about his medications and his greatest concern in administering them.

44. Which of the following statements **BEST** describes the learner in cognitive theory? The learner needs to
    A. be cognitively prepared to receive information and aware of the education session starting.
    B. recognize how information is used and why it is important to pay attention.
    C. show interest in the topic and be ready to learn.
    D. receive and process information before demonstrating understanding.

45. A patient presents with a history of diabetes and a new diagnosis of heart disease. The patient does not speak English and an interpreter will be present for patient education performed by the nurse care coordinator. Which of the following questions contain language that should be **AVOIDED,** as it is challenging to interpret?
    A. Have you felt blue since your hospitalization?
    B. How many times a day do you inject insulin?
    C. How has your life changed since your hospitalization?
    D. How often do you test your blood sugar?

46. Which of the following is an unacceptable method for working with an interpreter?
    A. Speak directly to the patient, not the interpreter.
    B. Speak directly to the interpreter.
    C. Verify patient understanding by asking the patient to explain in his or her own words, working with an interpreter.
    D. Allow sufficient time for the interaction.

47. Which example illustrates collaboration and teamwork required for successful engagement of patients and families in care?
    A. Setting the expectation that the patient's family and health care team work together toward a specific goal for the patient.
    B. Using team huddles and care conferences only when specific issues impacting patient outcome are identified.
    C. Determining resources within health care interprofessional teams to decrease cost.
    D. Coordinating the health care team to target the same health literacy level and education.

48. A patient with heart failure was admitted to the hospital with symptoms of difficulty breathing and a five-pound weight gain over 24 hours prior to admission. The patient was identified as one who would benefit from nursing care coordination. The nurse care coordinator from the cardiology clinic was contacted to meet with the patient prior to his discharge. Which of the following statements provides the elements of successful engagement for the patient and the patient's family to achieve success in management of his health care over time? The patient and family
    A. know the various roles of the team, partner with the team in setting goals, and make decisions about treatment in collaboration with the team.
    B. are compliant with the discharge plan, openly voice concerns, and know the professional to contact to get issues addressed.
    C. will report potential safety problems with medications, openly voice concerns, and know the professional to contact for questions.
    D. are comfortable communicating with the team, know the titles of the various team members, and openly voice concerns.

49. Which of the following statements identifies the nurse care coordinator's knowledge, skill, and attitude for competency in patient-centered care planning?
    A. Seeks to understand the values of the patient and family, elicits the patient values and preferences, and is flexible to solve problems with a commitment to the patient and family.
    B. Identifies components of a coordinated, integrated plan of care; uses a variety of evidence-based clinical care; and values continuous improvement of own conflict resolution skills.
    C. Seeks to assess physical, psychological, emotional, and other barriers to learning; provides patient-centered care with respect; and identifies one's own attitude concerning support of family members.
    D. Identifies support found through involvement of family and friends, uses motivational interviewing, and values the need to continuously improve one's own clinical practice.

50. Which of the following **BEST** illustrates the definition of patient education?
    A. The process of influencing health behavior and producing change.
    B. Any combination of planned learning experiences provided to individuals (and groups) to provide thoughts and information about health conditions.
    C. The process to engage individuals to take action in making changes about their health.
    D. A four-stage process for the patient to develop their skills and confidence in self-care.

51. Which of the following provides reliability in evaluating health information?
    A. Determining the authorship or sponsorship of the material.
    B. Offering the patient and family choices for the medium they prefer.
    C. Confirming the patient understands the material.
    D. Choosing material with illustrations for improved patient comprehension.

52. The health care team has been working with a patient over the past year to foster self-management skills. The five core self-management skills include problem solving, decision-making, and which of the following?
    A. Using resources, partnerships, and taking action.
    B. Care planning, partnerships, and taking action.
    C. Care planning, using resources, and taking action.
    D. Using resources, partnerships and care planning.

53. Which of the following statements **BEST** illustrates the competency of a nurse care coordinator for education and engagement of patients and families for planning care?
    A. Defines the differences between information, communication, and education; assesses the patient and family for readiness to learn; and creates an environment of communication and questioning that empowers the patient/family to engage in care.
    B. Coordinates the provision of patient education across the team, identifies a primary support person(s) for the patient, and values the need for continuous improvement in clinical practice.
    C. Identifies the appropriate approach to teaching after evaluating the patient's health literacy; assesses the patient's cognition, aptitude, and readiness to learn; and values evidence-based teaching techniques.
    D. Examines common barriers to active involvement of patients in their own health care processes, develops patient/family/caregiver ability to engage in decision-making, and values the importance of reading relevant professional journals regularly.

54. Which of the following methods would be best for the nurse care coordinator to use to facilitate learning?
    A. Use group competitive spirit to encourage active learning.
    B. Use word of mouth to create interest in a topic.
    C. Present information in short manageable sections.
    D. Encourage patients to explore Internet sites and critique findings.

55. A patient with chronic renal failure has been on peritoneal dialysis for the past year and is excited to attend a family wedding. The patient does not want to do her peritoneal dialysis because she must travel out of state for the wedding. Which of the following statements conveys the nurse care coordinator's attitude necessary for patient-centered planning?
    A. Seeks to understand the values of the patient and family, elicits the patient's values and preferences, and is flexible in assisting with problem solving with a commitment to the patient and family.
    B. Identifies components of a coordinated, integrated plan of care; uses a variety of evidence-based clinical care interventions; and values continuous improvement of own conflict resolution skills.
    C. Seeks to assess physical, psychological, emotional, and other barriers to learning; provides patient-centered care with respect; and identifies one's own attitude concerning support of family members.
    D. Uses evidence-based clinical plan, is flexible in assisting with problem-solving, and evaluates its effectiveness.

56. Clark Honas has come to the clinic today accompanied by his wife. Mrs. Honas informs the nurse care coordinator that her husband drinks alcohol to excess, has not told his provider, and she is concerned for his welfare. In receiving this information, what does the nurse care coordinator need to consider in assimilating the principles of care coordination and transition management (CCTM)?
    A. When conflict occurs, the nurse care coordinator must recognize boundaries, tension, shared decision-making, and empowerment of patients and families.
    B. Information disclosed by the patient's wife should be dismissed and not shared with other health care team members.
    C. The nurse care coordinator should inform the health care team about Mr. Honas's excessive alcohol intake.
    D. The nurse care coordinator should provide Mr. Honas with information about Alcoholics Anonymous.

57. Which of the following are the National Patient Safety Foundation's "Ask Me 3" questions that a patient is encouraged to ask a provider?
    A. What will my insurance cover? Will I have help? Will I have resources?
    B. Is my provider qualified? Is this covered by insurance? Will this be manageable?
    C. What will this cost? Where will I go? Who is here to help?
    D. What is my main problem? What do I need to do? Why is it important for me to do this?

58. The primary care clinic nursing staff is concerned about the patient education materials that are available in the waiting room. Which is the **BEST** method for the nurse care coordinator to evaluate patient education materials? Determine if the material…
    A. is based on evidence, can be reproduced in black and white to decrease copying costs, and contains references to websites.
    B. is based on evidence, contains a current publication date, and authorship indicates an authoritative source.
    C. contains a current publication date, contains non-biased information, and is written at the 5th grade reading level.
    D. contains a current publication date, contains non-biased information, and is available in multiple languages.

59. A nurse care coordinator is working in the OB-GYN clinic. A 26-year-old, prima gravida, is 8-weeks pregnant and asks for recommendations for a phone or computer application ("app") to use during her pregnancy. Which of the following is an appropriate response from the nurse care coordinator about technology in health care? The nurse care coordinator
    A. should refrain from recommending a specific app.
    B. is aware mobile technology and Cloud computing play a major role in care coordination and transition management.
    C. should ask the patient to identify several apps and the nurse care coordinator can review them and make a recommendation.
    D. is aware it is inappropriate to recommend pregnancy apps for the patient.

60. The American Nurses Association (2010) defines nursing informatics as a specialty that integrates nursing science, computer science, and which of the following?
    A. Health information technology.
    B. Computer programs.
    C. Information science.
    D. Health records.

61. Which of the following demonstrates how health information technology supports activities related to care coordination?
    A. Facilitating transfer of information, improving outcomes of care for high-risk populations, and managing data.
    B. Providing a complete record of care for all parties to access simultaneously, managing data, and mitigating error.
    C. Facilitating transfer of information, enabling communication between parties in different locations, and providing real-time decision support.
    D. Providing a complete record of care for all parties to access simultaneously, improving outcomes of care for high-risk populations, and mitigating error.

62. The nurse care coordinator is reviewing the care of a patient referred for care coordination. Which of the following demonstrates the nurse care coordinator's ability to use health information technology to support care coordination activities? The nurse care coordinator
    A. is able to navigate the EHR to review the patient's plan of care.
    B. uses performance improvement tools to assess use of technology to improve care.
    C. values systems thinking and the use of health information technology to improve care.
    D. uses data and electronic reports to improve coordination of care.

63. The nurse care coordinator is reviewing a report of patients scheduled to come into the clinic in the upcoming week. Which of the following statements is **MOST** supportive of health information technology for the RN-CCTM Model?
    A. The report enables the nurse care coordinator to proactively identify patients needing a pneumococcal vaccine.
    B. Use of health information technology has the potential to reduce cost and improve outcomes for all populations in all health settings.
    C. The use of reports is standard for all patients receiving care coordination.
    D. Health information technology reduces the workload of the nurse care coordinator to review each patient's record.

64. The nursing team of the surgical clinic meets to review a report of patients who are receiving pre-surgical teaching. The report includes the following information: patient's name, age, gender, diagnosis(es), and co-morbidities. Since the report was implemented, the nurse care coordinators discovered they are better prepared to anticipate patient concerns about their surgery. Which of these statements **BEST** reflects how the use of this type of report supports coordination in patient care?
    A. The nurse care coordinators can proactively develop a plan for patient education.
    B. The report targets patients needing pre-surgical teaching and the nursing staff can determine which nurse care coordinators should be assigned to provide teaching.
    C. The nurse care coordinators are able to print specific patient education handouts before the patient arrives for the appointment.
    D. The nurse care coordinators can explain to the patient who the surgical team members will be on the day of their surgery.

65. The Adult Primary Care Medicine Clinic utilizes a report for identifying all patients needing a pneumococcal vaccine. Since the report was implemented several years ago, the clinic's percentage rate of patients who are 65 years and older receiving the pneumococcal vaccine has increased steadily. Which of the following statements describes the use of information and technology as decision-support tools?
    A. They are used with critical thinking and critical judgment.
    B. They can be used to dictate practice.
    C. They can replace the need for providers to write orders for preventive care activities.
    D. They can be used to enhance communication within the clinical team.

66. The Information Technology Department will integrate information from the EHR, Internet, and health information exchange to identify high-risk diabetic patients for the nurse care coordinator. Which of the following statements describes how this information about the various health IT solutions may be used for the new program? This information will be used to…
    A. categorize patients at high and low risk for diabetic complications.
    B. sort patient demographics, age, and education level.
    C. stratify patients into insurance coverage, risk, and compliance categories.
    D. communicate, manage knowledge, mitigate error, and support decision-making.

67. Health information technology supports patient safety in which of the following ways?
    A. Allows identification of data to be accessed for a limited period of time.
    B. Allows capture of data to help nurse care coordinators monitor cost and compliance.
    C. Supports evaluation of population health outcomes to ensure patients receive appropriate and timely care.
    D. Supports team collaboration and provides alerts when pertinent information is missing when the patient transitions from one setting to another.

68. The Pediatric Clinic uses a documentation system that asks for input on the child's date of birth, weight, immunization history, and other pertinent facts. An algorithm is used to provide a recommendation for the next scheduled immunization. What type of system is capable of providing this recommendation?
    A. Decision support system.
    B. Database system.
    C. Information seeking system.
    D. Health care system.

69. Which of the following is an example of *syndromic surveillance*?
    A. Using health information from the Internet for surveillance of population outbreaks.
    B. Tracking data of patient symptoms that signal a potential population outbreak that would warrant further response.
    C. Targeting the investigation of potential population outbreaks.
    D. Using a system capable of identifying diagnoses that have clustered in specific geographic areas for targeted intervention.

70. Which of these is an example of an element of evidence-based decision support in care coordination?
    A. Institutional support for prioritization of evidence for care coordination.
    B. An interprofessional team focused on improving reimbursement for care transitions.
    C. Standardized pathways that highlight key medical and medication changes, follow-up and self-management instructions, and tests.
    D. Reports that inform the team and front-line workers of errors of omission from the standardized pathways for improvement.

Questions 71-72 refer to the following patient case.

The mother of a 10-year-old girl diagnosed with cerebral palsy calls the nurse care coordinator in the outpatient primary care clinic. She discusses her daughter's increased difficulty ambulating at school with her new orthotics and wonders if she needs to be evaluated for additional physical therapy.

71. Which of the following responses **BEST** demonstrates the value of the patient and family as members of the health care team?
    A. Next week, when the doctor returns to the office, I will have him call you with a plan.
    B. I will make an appointment for your daughter to be seen by a physical therapist.
    C. I will communicate your concerns and thoughts to the team and will get back to you later today.
    D. I will make an appointment for your daughter to be seen by the doctor in the primary care clinic.

72. The nurse care coordinator communicates the mother's observations and concerns to the other members of the interprofessional team and all agree further evaluation and referral to the physical therapist is warranted. Which is the **MOST** effective way for the nurse care coordinator to effectively facilitate communication of the team's thoughts to the mother?
    A. Call the mother with a date and time for an appointment with the physical therapist.
    B. Mail a summary of the health care team's discussion to the mother for review.
    C. Call the mother to see if she would like to meet in-person with the care coordinator to discuss the team's thoughts.
    D. E-mail the mother a summary of the team's thoughts and an appointment with a physical therapist.

Questions 73-75 refer to the following patient case.

Carlos Casper, 17-years-old, sustained a traumatic brain injury with residual memory loss. He and his parents meet with his care team to review his personal action plan to determine his level of progress toward his goals. Carlos states he continues to forget to wear his helmet when riding his bicycle.

73. The nurse care coordinator provides specific information about the potential health risks of not wearing a helmet to encourage a change in behavior. This is an example of which of the Five A's Change Concept?
    A. Assess.
    B. Assist.
    C. Advise.
    D. Arrange.

74. Carlos states he never falls off his bike and he doesn't think he needs to wear his helmet all of the time just because of his brain injury. Which phase of change is Carlos depicting by this statement?
    A. Pre-contemplation.
    B. Contemplation.
    C. Preparation.
    D. Action.

75. The nurse care coordinator works with Carlos to develop goals around wearing his helmet when he rides his bike. Carlos states he will have his parents help him document each time he wears his helmet. This is an example of which part of his SMART goal?
    A. Attainable.
    B. Specific.
    C. Timely.
    D. Measurable.

Questions 76-78 refer to the following patient case.

Ben Kline, a 15-year-old with spina bifida, receives primary care in the only clinic available in his rural community.

76. As the nurse care coordinator in the clinic, which of the following can be used to guide care coordination needs around effective communication through the use of health information technology (HIT)?
    A. National Quality Strategy.
    B. Technology Informatics Guiding Education Reform.
    C. Agency for Healthcare Research and Quality.
    D. Technology for Economic and Clinical Health.

77. The nurse care coordinator for Ben is aware care coordination integrates care across the continuum including what dimensions of information?
    A. Needs, experiences, and health care conditions.
    B. Needs, resources, and education.
    C. Required services, access to funding, and education.
    D. Required services, access to funding, and location.

78. As the nurse care coordinator and pivotal member of the health care team, how would one use the EHR to aid in the ongoing coordination of Ben's specialty care needs? Share information…
    A. within and outside of the practice, integrating specialty care.
    B. with caution and filtering, integrating selective care.
    C. with caution and filtering, selecting special care.
    D. share information within the practice to aim for selective care.

79. The Health Information Technology for Economic and Clinical Health Act of 2009 adopted which of the following for certified EHRs to improve quality and reduce health care costs through financial incentives?
    A. Meaningful use.
    B. Personal health records.
    C. Mobile technology.
    D. Nursing informatics.

80. Coordination of care and population health management are systems dependent on which of the following for the transfer of information and communication?
    A. Personal health record (PHR).
    B. Health information technology (HIT).
    C. Electronic health record (EHR).
    D. Health information exchange (HIE).

81. What statement **BEST** describes the goal of population health management (PHM)?
    A. Keeping a population as healthy as possible.
    B. Tracking low-risk patients in a population to ensure health.
    C. Modifying life factors that exacerbate illnesses.
    D. Increasing the life expectancy of a selected population.

82. What is the characteristic that **MOST** accurately describes a necessary component in PHM?
    A. Providing continuous care by the same nurses through hospitalization.
    B. Enhancing access to hospitals and EDs.
    C. Using interprofessional care teams.
    D. Encouraging individual provider management of a population's wellness.

83. A nurse care coordinator uses the Population Health Management Process to review and organize patients in a family practice clinic. What is the nurse care coordinator's **FIRST** step to organize the family practice clinic?
    A. Delivery of patient-centered interventions.
    B. Identification of a population to monitor and track.
    C. Focus on health behavior and lifestyle changes.
    D. Initiating health risk management.

84. Which of the following is an example of an element of Wagner's Chronic Care Model (1998) that guides processes to improve chronic illness care?
    A. Patient self-management organized and based in local hospitals.
    B. Enhanced provider education based on professional proclivities and skills.
    C. Team functioning organized around standard office hours and patient reminders.
    D. Enhanced information systems to facilitate development of tracking systems.

85. What is the **MOST** effective method of data collection to track and monitor the health of high-risk patients and identify groups for care coordination?
    A. Patient and/or caregiver-reported data.
    B. Registry lists from health plans.
    C. Multiple data source predictive analytics.
    D. Claims data from clinic and health plans.

86. What is the **BEST** example of a subpopulation that might benefit from additional CCTM services while demonstrating an effective use of population management resources?
    A. Patients needing colorectal screening who are 50 years of age and older.
    B. Diabetic patients with A1Cs indicating risk for diabetes.
    C. Patients who received reminders of follow-up visits with primary care provider (PCP).
    D. Patients over 40 receiving nutritional education from a dietician.

87. The **MOST** efficient method for the nurse care coordinator to stratify a practice's patients into populations needing care coordination is to stratify by
    A. disease diagnosis.
    B. their risk of getting sick or sicker.
    C. exclusion of healthy people in the practice.
    D. daily by care team huddles.

88. Which of the following processes will be the **MOST** effective for the nurse care coordinator to address with the aim of closing gaps in care for preventive services and chronic condition management?
    A. Simplify care by reviewing charts to look for overdue mammograms and colorectal screening.
    D. Initiate care by arranging appointments for selected patients with phone notification of the upcoming visit.
    C. Support care by sending brief education modules regularly to enhance patient and family experience with the practice.
    D. Facilitate care by utilization of a hospital discharge registry to ensure continuity with the transition across the health care continuum.

89. Which example **BEST** demonstrates the concept of team-based interventions for PHM in an outpatient setting?
    A. Small teams may include a PCP and a receptionist/secretary for effective utilization of resources.
    B. Physician providers focus on each area and phase of patient care delivery to ensure improved outcomes for delivery of quality care.
    C. Larger teams may have health coaches, pharmacists, and therapists to ensure delivery of care that requires staff and resources beyond what individual primary care physicians can provide.
    D. Clinic managers schedule medical assistants to relieve receptionists for continuity of workflow and information management throughout the work day.

90. What is a **MAJOR** responsibility of the nurse care coordinator as a member of a CCTM team?
    A. Attending or leading daily huddles on the day of the office visit to discuss needed patient interventions.
    B. Reviewing charts for pre-visit within 2 months before potential visits.
    C. Categorizing patients with one or fewer chronic conditions in a large practice with many patients identified as high-risk.
    D. Managing a caseload of up to 15,000 Medicare patients in a practice.

91. What statement is the **BEST** example of how EHRs are utilized by a CCTM team to share information with the aim of improving population health?
    A. Billing information for reviewing patient financial needs.
    B. Direct relief of physical discomfort for both high and low-risk populations.
    C. Communicate knowledge gained from needs assessment from different domains of care.
    D. Patient engagement and enhancement of patient and family care experiences.

92. How can the nurse care coordinator use the health plan registry to identify patients and manage outcomes?
    A. Prioritize patients with high-risk clinical conditions, serious unmet clinical need for outreach, and intervention to manage outcomes.
    B. Identify patients who are frequent users of high-cost health care services and prioritize patients with health plan billing issues.
    C. Identify patients at risk due to family chronic disease, users of high-cost services, and prioritize appointment management.
    D. Prioritize patients who missed their most recent PCP appointment, have unmet billing needs, and have abnormal lab values.

Questions 93-98 refer to the following patient case.

Tim Sea is 67-years-old with a history of smoking and Type 2 diabetes managed with an oral hypoglycemic. Mr. Sea was discharged recently from the hospital with a new diagnosis of moderate-to-severe COPD. Mr. Sea has a history of missed appointments with his PCP, and has identified economic hardship with paying his co-pay. The nurse care coordinator has been working with Mr. Sea to consider a smoking cessation program. Eight months before this hospital admission the nurse care coordinator called Mr. Sea by phone following a missed appointment. Mr. Sea reported he is not interested in stopping his smoking habit ("I enjoy it too much") but agreed he would cut back for the financial savings. Following this hospital discharge, Mr. Sea attended his appointment with his PCP.

93. What concept of informatics does the nurse care coordinator apply to address Mr. Sea's missed appointment history?
    A. Registries are important tools to monitor patients for compliance with daily health habits and assist with health promotion.
    B. Registries are important tools to prioritize patients for gaps in care and lack of post-discharge follow-up.
    C. Registries are tools to manage post-discharge follow-up and medication management.
    D. Registries are important tools to support health promotion behavior.

94. What is the **MOST** appropriate statement regarding the nurse care coordinator's telephone outreach with Mr. Sea?
    A. The nurse care coordinator knows how to utilize telephone outreach and locate patients who miss appointments.
    B. The telephone outreach demonstrated the nurse care coordinator's knowledge of how difficult smoking cessation programs can be.
    C. The telephone outreach demonstrated the impact of engagement on health outcomes and how patients demonstrate better outcomes when they collaborate with providers.
    D. The nurse care coordinator utilized telephone outreach to manage a noncompliant patient and mitigate complications of this noncompliance.

95. Which of the project Better Outcomes by Optimizing Safe Transitions (BOOST) 8Ps Risk Assessment Tool factors was identified as a potential factor leading to Mr. Sea's unfavorable outcomes after hospital discharge?
    A. "Problem" medications.
    B. Lack of "primary care."
    C. "Principle" diagnosis.
    D. Lack of "palliative" care.

96. What is the **MOST** applicable way for the nurse care coordinator to assist Mr. Sea in managing his transition of care?
    A. Obtain objective and subjective data pertaining to Mr. Sea's concerns about his new diagnosis.
    B. Collect subjective data from Mr. Sea's family regarding his progress.
    C. Collect objective lab results of previous PCP appointments for review.
    D. Delegate the medical assistant to obtain objective data with an outreach call and appointment scheduling.

97. Which tool can the nurse care coordinator use to assess Mr. Sea's level of engagement with his care?
    A. Patient activation measure (PAM).
    B. Electronic health record (EHR).
    C. Patient health management (PHM).
    D. Health information technology (HIT).

98. The nurse care coordinator met with Mr. Sea before his PCP appointment. During the visit, Mr. Sea expressed the feeling of being overwhelmed. After listening to Mr. Sea, what is the **BEST** recommendation to assist the nurse care coordinator in Mr. Sea's care management?
    A. Remember the principles of motivational interviewing and appropriate actions.
    B. Consider the relationship between patient activation measure and disease burden.
    C. Be aware of burden of chronic disease management in a complex health care system.
    D. Maintain vigilant surveillance of indicators leading to noncompliance and poor disease management.

Questions 99-100 refer to the following patient case.

A nurse care coordinator is newly hired at a clinic that serves the health care needs of a population of single male and female military recruits. The average age is 18-20, and all patients are without chronic health conditions.

99. What initial action can the nurse care coordinator take to **BEST** serve this healthy population?
    A. Implement a schedule of running for all clinic staff to demonstrate to the recruits the clinic staff members' commitment to staying fit, design and post information charts for healthy exercise, and establish a system to display workout accomplishments of clinic staff.
    B. Schedule interviews with each soldier to establish a provider relationship and develop an understanding of the needs of every soldier who will utilize the clinic.
    C. Review the family history of the soldiers assigned to the clinic and develop classes using evidence-based research to target potential diseases they may face in the future.
    D. Research evidence-based preventive practice in this age group, review data from EHRs, and interview the military base leaders to assess where to target preventive care.

100. The nurse care coordinator identifies evidence-based Centers for Disease Control and Prevention (CDC) immunization recommendations for this age group to include Tdap or Td, flu vaccines, and which of the following immunizations?
    A. Human papillomavirus (HPV) and meningococcal for both female and male recruits.
    B. HPV vaccine for female recruits only, and meningococcal for both male and female recruits.
    C. Meningococcal for female recruits and measles, mumps, and rubella (MMR) for male recruits.
    D. MMR for both male and female recruits and HPV for female recruits only.

101. When building a registry of patients for PHM at the practice setting level, what is the most comprehensive data set to begin building the registry?
    A. List of patients who contact the health care delivery system through phone calls and office visits.
    B. Reports generated that identify alerts generated by the EHR and emails.
    C. Information identifying health plan eligibility and administrative data on the assigned patient subpopulation.
    D. Listserv of patients who have not had an office visit in the last year.

102. If the nurse care coordinator is working with a population of patients diagnosed with epilepsy, which of the following outcome measures would be tracked for identifying patients who are high risk?
    A. Number of medications, number of phone calls to office, number of caregivers involved in care, and number of missed appointments.
    B. Income level, distance of residence from office, public transportation use, and number of seizures.
    C. Number of specialists involved in care, number of diagnoses on problem list, number of missed appointments.
    D. Number of seizures, number of ED visits, and number of missed days at school or work since last office visit.

103. What cornerstone of the Population Health Management Model sets the model apart from a traditional disease management program?
    A. Proactive identification and closure of gaps in care.
    B. Education for self-management and health promotion.
    C. Development of cultural competence and cultural safety.
    D. Utilization of outreach and reminders for patient communication.

104. What is the goal of a nurse care coordinator when promoting patient engagement?
    A. Achieving higher levels of action on the part of patient to self-manage care.
    B. Receiving fewer phone calls between visits for issues and concerns.
    C. Promoting adherence to the plan of care and better outcomes.
    D. Facilitating connection between the patient and community advocacy groups.

105. The nurse care coordinator is caring for a group of pediatric patients with Type 2 diabetes. After determining the level of care coordination required through risk stratification, what is the foundation of the care plan developed by the nurse care coordinator?
    A. Community support utilizing recommendations from lay-led advocacy groups for people with diabetes.
    B. Evidence-based measures, such as the standards of care outlined by the American Diabetes Association.
    C. Health literacy level of the patient and education from national diabetes advocacy groups.
    D. Hospital Consumer Assessment of Healthcare Providers and Systems (HCAHPS) survey patient engagement measures and apply findings to select compatible provider.

106. How does the nurse care coordinator utilize work reminders when working with an established patient who is diagnosed with epilepsy?
    A. Notify primary care provider when patient is hospitalized.
    B. Track and promote adherence to preventive screenings, tests, and exams.
    C. Track and document content of incoming and outgoing phone calls for cross-continuum communication.
    D. Remind patient to participate in community epilepsy advocacy group events.

107. Which of the following is an example of a modality for preventive care management, where the nurse care coordinator incorporates automated systems in the care plan to promote adherence to wellness and preventive care interventions?
    A. Mailing a reminder letter for mammogram screening, automatically generated by the EHR.
    B. Reminding the patient at discharge from the office visit to schedule annual preventive appointments.
    C. Providing the patient with a flyer advertising an upcoming health fair with blood pressure screening.
    D. Keeping a log of patients to call when flu season begins to promote immunization against the flu.

108. When the nurse care coordinator works with a growing group of pediatric patients with precocious puberty receiving surgically implanted medication to manage the condition. What is the **BEST** action to coordinate the care for this population?
    A. Develop an Excel worksheet to track care milestones and outcomes.
    B. Create a folder on a shared drive to promote communication among the caregivers.
    C. Document all of the care coordination in the outpatient EHR.
    D. Collaborate with the informatics team to develop a registry in the EHR.

109. What is the **PRIMARY** critical function of the decision-support tools in the EHR that are established by the nurse care coordinator?
    A. Health education at the appropriate literacy level.
    B. Prevention, safety, and utilization alerts.
    C. List of resources tailored to the age and primary diagnosis of the patient.
    D. Reminder calls for upcoming scheduled appointments.

110. When a nurse care coordinator is working with the diabetes population and is vested in making sure the impact of CCTM is equitable across socioeconomic groups. What does the nurse care coordinator monitor to ensure equitable care between the commercially insured patients vs. government-insured patients?
    A. Number of patients who access group self-management education classes.
    B. Number of work reminders generated for these patients.
    C. Normal lab results for the active patients.
    D. Length of office visit for these patients.

111. To describe the efficacy of PHM for a set of patients with diabetes, what is an important outcome to measure and track?
    A. Electronic communications that have no response.
    B. Community faith group participation.
    C. Missed days from school or work in the last year.
    D. Work or school performance.

112. Systems that manage and track information related to population health should include what elements to provide comprehensive evaluation of outcomes?
    A. Claims data, hospital admission and visit data, and EHR clinical value data.
    B. Cycle time data, call volume data, and Grade of Service (GOS).
    C. Budget variance data, slot utilization data, and Time To Next Available (TTNA).
    D. Patient experience data, self-reported social media use, and number of missed medication doses.

113. What act or organization, which is part of the American Recovery and Reinvestment Act of 2009 (ARRA), widens the scope of privacy and security protections available under Health Insurance Portability and Accountability Act (HIPAA), increases the potential legal liability for noncompliance, and provides for more enforcement of HIPAA rules?
    A. Healthcare Information and Management System Society (HIMSS).
    B. Health Information Technology for Economic and Clinical Health Act (HITECH).
    C. National Committee for Quality Assurance Patient Centered Medical Home Act (NCQA PCMH).
    D. Business Associate Agreement Act (BAA).

114. What is the one important development in telehealth with implications for the nurse care coordinator that impacts the mobilization of health care information electronically across organizations within a region, community, or a hospital system?
    A. Health Insurance Portability and Accountability Act (HIPAA).
    B. Electronic health record (EHR).
    C. Business Associate Agreement (BAA).
    D. Health information exchange (HIE).

115. What is defined as the use of information and technology to communicate, manage knowledge, mitigate error, and support decision-making?
    A. Evidenced-based practice.
    B. Quality improvement.
    C. Informatics.
    D. Safety.

116. What is defined as the use of data to monitor the outcomes of care processes and use of methods to design and test changes with the goal of optimizing the quality and safety of health care systems?
    A. Evidence-based practice.
    B. Quality improvement.
    C. Informatics.
    D. Safety.

117. When the nurse care coordinator practices patient-centered care within a population health management framework, what does the nurse care coordinator assess as possible obstacles to compliance?
    A. Gaps in care.
    B. Barriers to care.
    C. Decisional conflict.
    D. Value of non-consensus.

118. What is the nurse care coordinator assessing when evaluating the degree to which the patient has the capacity to obtain, process, and understand basic health information and services needed to make appropriate health decisions?
    A. Cultural diversity.
    B. Social background.
    C. Health care equity.
    D. Health literacy.

119. What are the systematically developed statements that the nurse care coordinator uses to assist provider and patient decisions about appropriate health care for specific circumstances?
    A. Consensus reports.
    B. Clinical practice guidelines.
    C. Standard operating procedures.
    D. Protocol pathways.

120. To understand the efficacy of PHM with regard to outcomes, what is important to compare performance against?
    A. Population-relevant benchmarks.
    B. Disease-specific registry data.
    C. Consensus statement recommendations.
    D. Previous outcome data.

121. The nurse care coordinator prepares for care planning and needs assessment for a patient by reviewing the chart and identifying the following: the patient is recently unemployed, is returning for findings related to biopsy results, and has no family or next of kin of record. The nurse care coordinator assesses the patient for depression by choosing which of the following assessment tools?
    A. Functional Assessment.
    B. Cage and Cage-AID.
    C. Psychosocial Assessment.
    D. Mini-Cog.

122. Mark Johnson has an appointment for his annual physical exam. Mrs. Johnson, his wife, accompanies him to the appointment. Mrs. Johnson shares with the nurse care coordinator that she is unable to keep her own appointments for her health care, she often feels disconnected from friends and family, and she has difficulty making ends meet with their fixed incomes. Why might the nurse care coordinator administer the Modified Caregiver Strain Index assessment?
    A. To identify appropriate interventions needed to help Mrs. Johnson.
    B. To ask Mrs. Johnson about sources of funding needed to provide assistance.
    C. To obtain information necessary to refer to a financial counselor.
    D. To ask Mrs. Johnson about other family members who might support their needs.

Questions 123-125 refer to the following patient case.

The nurse care coordinator prepares for scheduled patient visits for the following Monday.

123. The nurse care coordinator uses the EHR to identify gaps in care and to conduct pre-visit chart reviews. Choose the **BEST** action appropriate during this early phase of the patient assessment.
    A. Ask the front desk clerk to verify demographic information.
    B. Consult the provider about his or her schedule.
    C. Question the patient's insurance coverage.
    D. Question if medications are up to date (expired or need refill).

124. Based on the patient's age, gender, and current diagnoses, which preventive health recommendations might the nurse care coordinator make in planning for the visit?
    A. Administration of a cognitive assessment.
    B. Updates to care plan.
    C. Specialist appointments for potential exacerbations of current conditions.
    D. Screenings and/or tests outstanding or missing.

125. Which action **BEST** demonstrates the nurse care coordinator understands the visit planning process?
    A. Review missing x-rays, labs, referrals, and immunizations with PCP prior to visit, so orders can be obtained.
    B. Meet with the pharmacist to discuss the patient's home medications.
    C. Contact the patient at home to schedule a planned visit.
    D. Contact the patient's next of kin of record to plan for a needs assessment.

Questions 126 and 127 refer to the following patient case.

The nurse care coordinator is ready to develop the patient-centered care plans for scheduled patients. Proactively, the nurse care coordinator identifies all at-risk patients first.

126. The nurse care coordinator identifies patients at-risk by selecting which of the following strategies?
    A. Chronic disease-based models, such as diabetes-specific models.
    B. Analytic software tools, such as Domo and SPSS.
    C. Low-risk patients with acute illnesses, under 40, with short hospital stays.
    D. Risk stratification for in-hospital mortality models.

127. During the chart review, the nurse care coordinator identifies a 65-year-old diabetic patient with an HbA1c of 9.3 and Stage 2 hypertension. The PCP visit is a follow-up to a recent hospital discharge for a hyperglycemic episode. The nurse care coordinator calls the patient for intake and assessment. What is the **BEST** action of the nurse care coordinator during the call?
    A. Tell the patient noncompliance with medication and the diet that the provider has prescribed will further complicate the disease.
    B. Explain that the nurse care coordinator is available to help with medications, disease-specific questions, transportation, and to coordinate care overall.
    C. Explain why certain questions cannot be answered over the phone and arrange for an office visit with the nurse care coordinator, aside from a provider visit.
    D. Verify insurance coverage and drug plan formulary for best support of the plan at the lowest out-of-pocket expense for the patient.

128. A patient tells the nurse care coordinator, "I was frightened when my son had to call the ambulance because I was vomiting and had severe stomach pain! It turns out when I arrived to the ER my blood sugar was 700! I really learned my lesson. I am ready to start eating better. What can I do?" What should the nurse care coordinator use to demonstrate the patient is progressing through stages of change?
    A. Sustain talk.
    B. Behavioral theory.
    C. Change talk.
    D. Resistance talk.

129. What attitude toward change is the counseling method Motivational Interviewing used to address?
    A. Worries.
    B. Apprehension.
    C. Acceptance.
    D. Ambivalence.

130. The nurse care coordinator uses skillful clinical communication when discussing lifestyle changes with James McKinley, a patient with diabetes mellitus. How would the nurse care coordinator build rapport with the patient?
    A. Set goals for the series of educational encounters.
    B. Ask open-ended questions and support his decision-making.
    C. Provide direct advice about sick day care and how to adjust his diet and medication regimen.
    D. Help Mr. McKinley to identify barriers to his compliance with the care plan.

Questions 131 and 132 refer to the following patient case.

131. Tom Stark presents to his primary care provider for follow-up for nutrition management and weight reduction. Mr. Stark and the nurse care coordinator discuss goals agreeable to Mr. Stark. Which of these statements by Mr. Stark would **BEST** be supported by the nurse care coordinator because it reflects patient-driven goal setting?
    A. "The doctor wants me to exercise three times a week."
    B. "I should reduce my intake of soda and sugar, according to the dietitian."
    C. "I know that I can add more fruits and vegetables to my diet."
    D. "I know I should consider broiling instead of frying meats, fish, and poultry."

132. Mr. Stark and the nurse care coordinator set patient-centered goals during his visit. In demonstrating competency in patient education, what should the nurse care coordinator ensure the patient receives before he departs?
    A. Information about weight-reduction programs in the community.
    B. Material about nutrition that is based on his limited literacy.
    C. Educational material about pre-diabetes risks.
    D. A DVD about weight management for him to review at home before the next visit.

133. Which term is used to describe activities or treatments that are based on the results of clinical research?
    A. Evidence-based practice.
    B. Clinical guideline.
    C. Standard protocol.
    D. Scientific method.

134. The nurse care coordinator works collaboratively with patients and providers to achieve quality improvements in health care through breast cancer screening, colorectal screening, and Chlamydia screening. The nurse care coordinator applies knowledge of these quality improvement measures by interpreting results from which of the following tools?
    A. Patients at Risk for Re-hospitalization (PARR).
    B. Length of stay, acuity of admission, co-morbidity, and ED visits to identify patients with a high risk for readmission or death (LACE).
    C. Healthcare Effectiveness Data and Information Set (HEDIS™).
    D. Better Outcomes for Older Adults through Safe Transitions (BOOST).

135. The nurse care coordinator conducts a review of a patient's record for the need of care coordination related to the diagnosis of congestive heart failure, and reviews current treatment recommendations, prescribed medications, and hospital admissions. The nurse care coordinator might identify which of the following as a "red flag" when monitoring the patient's progress?
    A. Absence of pneumonia and influenza vaccination in the patient's history.
    B. Hospital readmissions, including all-cause 30-day readmissions.
    C. Missed physical therapy visits.
    D. Absence of a visit with a cardiologist in the last 6 months.

136. Which of the following demonstrates a barrier to patient engagement?
    A. Information learned on the Internet.
    B. Low health literacy (education).
    C. Patients talking to friends and relatives.
    D. Interest in homeopathic remedies.

137. The nurse care coordinator talks to a patient, Melvin Jackson, about his desire to manage his health and health care. The nurse care coordinator explains to Mr. Jackson the need to identify his knowledge and skill regarding his health. Which of the following is the **MOST** appropriate assessment tool for Mr. Jackson?
    A. Patient Health Questionnaire (PHQ).
    B. Get Up and Go Test.
    C. Patient Activation Measure (PAM).
    D. Clock Drawing Test.

138. Which of the following is a characteristic of motivational interviewing?
    A. Emotional.
    B. Helpful.
    C. Reflexive.
    D. Evocative.

Questions 139-142 refer to the following patient case.

Kathy Miller is a 56-year-old diagnosed with Type 2 diabetes, hypertension, hyperlipidemia, and obesity. She has been prescribed several oral medications and previously has received instruction in dietary measures to control her blood sugar and lipid levels. Ms. Miller's primary care provider has asked the nurse care coordinator to work with her to assist with improving her management of her chronic conditions.

139. At the first encounter, which of the following is the **PRIMARY** focus of the nurse care coordinator?
    A. Performing an assessment of Ms. Miller's medications and completing medication reconciliation with the prescribed medication list.
    B. Providing instructions on "sick day" care, when Ms. Miller's blood sugar and blood pressure may be more difficult to manage.
    C. Assessing Ms. Miller's understanding of her chronic conditions and how she manages them.
    D. Reviewing her complete medical history and assessing current symptoms and lab values.

140. Ms. Miller believes heredity is the cause of her metabolic disorders, and nothing she does will make a significant difference. What is the nurse care coordinator's **BEST** response?
    A. "Have you been down, depressed, or unhappy over the past 2 weeks?"
    B. "What members of your family had diabetes, high cholesterol, and hypertension?"
    C. "There are new medications that can better control your conditions than they probably had for your relatives in the past. Let's review your medications."
    D. "Heredity is one of many factors that contribute to these problems, but so is lifestyle. What are some of the things you are currently doing to manage them?"

141. After discussion, Ms. Miller believes reducing her intake of junk food would be an important change that she might be able to make. What is the nurse care coordinator's **BEST** response?
    A. Ask Ms. Miller for her weight goal.
    B. Inform Ms. Miller the primary care provider's goal for her is to get her HbA1c under 7.0.
    C. Ask Ms. Miller how important this change is for her, and specifically what will she do.
    D. Suggest she see a nutrition counselor.

142. The nurse care coordinator asks Ms. Miller what barriers she might face in reducing her intake of junk food. Ms. Miller states her whole family eats a lot of sweet and salty snacks and it will be hard for her to resist when she sees others eating these things that she likes. How should the nurse care coordinator support Ms. Miller's development of self-efficacy?
    A. Tell her to remove all snack food from the house.
    B. Explore how confident she is making the change and what might she do to improve her confidence.
    C. Ask her to bring her family to the next encounter so the barriers might be discussed together.
    D. Tell her how serious the consequences are for not making this change.

143. A nurse care coordinator telephones a patient following his visit to the ED the evening before. The patient is a smoker, has COPD, and a history of frequent ED visits. The nurse care coordinator learns the patient had run out of the prescribed inhaler, was coughing, and became increasingly short of breath (SOB). The patient states breathing treatments in the ED are effective for improving SOB. What is the **BEST** approach to support the patient's self-efficacy?
    A. Determine if there are barriers to using his prescribed medications effectively.
    B. Schedule him to see a pulmonologist to improve his COPD management plan.
    C. Schedule him for pulmonary function testing to assess the efficacy of bronchodilators.
    D. Explore his readiness to stop smoking.

144. Evidence supports motivational interviewing is an effective method of supporting self-regulation. Which of the following **BEST** describes motivational interviewing?
    A. Is effective with all patient populations.
    B. Uses peers as coaches, educators, and group facilitators.
    C. Uses communication techniques such as open-ended questions, affirmation, and reflection.
    D. Facilitates behavioral change through assessment, advice, agreement, assistance, and arrangement of follow-up.

145. Which of the following should the nurse care coordinator assess as a cognitive barrier to self-management?
    A. Physical changes that impact the patient's ability to be employed.
    B. Increased tension within the patient's family as the burden of his care becomes greater.
    C. Medication changes, including those that may be sedating.
    D. The patient expresses the desire to discuss end-of-life wishes.

Questions 146 and 147 refer to the following patient case.

Karen Frank is a 40-year-old with chronic, persistent asthma who presented to the primary care office for an urgent visit. She is short of breath and wheezing.

146. The provider prescribed a change in Ms. Frank's inhaler. The nurse care coordinator met with Ms. Frank and learned she is having some financial issues. What is the nurse care coordinator's next action?
    A. Approach the provider to prescribe a less costly inhaler.
    B. Refer Ms. Frank to a social worker to fully understand her financial barriers to care and options.
    C. Discuss with Ms. Frank what barriers to her self-care might be caused by her economic situation.
    D. Review the importance of filling the prescription for her maintenance inhaler, and not relying on her rescue inhaler.

147. In a follow-up call, the nurse care coordinator listens as Ms. Frank describes her improved symptoms, her self-satisfaction that she is using her maintenance inhaler daily, and that she has created a reminder system for herself. Ms. Frank is demonstrating which self-regulation skill?
    A. Goal-setting.
    B. Evaluation and tailoring.
    C. Development of an asthma action plan.
    D. Managing the emotional responses to her chronic condition.

148. The nurse care coordinator in a multispecialty office learns that Mark Major, a 35-year-old who is recovering from a motor vehicle accident, is drinking heavily every evening and now recognizes his drinking habit is a significant barrier to managing his health. He states he will quit his heavy drinking sometime in the next 6 months. What stage of readiness to change **BEST** describes Mr. Major's current state?
    A. Contemplative.
    B. Maintenance.
    C. Action.
    D. Pre-contemplative.

149. A patient is considering her self-management tasks and her confidence in the ability to make behavioral changes. What self-regulation skill describes the patient's behavior?
    A. Decision-making.
    B. Goal setting and self-monitoring.
    C. Reflective thinking.
    D. Development of an action plan.

150. Which of the following describes follow-up in support of a patient's self-management?
    A. Follow-up is most effective if performed by telephone.
    B. Follow-up should always be performed by a health professional team member rather than a peer coach.
    C. The value of follow-up is enhanced if it addresses the patient's data, progress toward goals, and barriers.
    D. Follow-up is ineffective in behavioral change for risk factor reduction, although it is effective for chronic condition self-management.

CCTM Domain V: Teamwork and Interprofessional Collaboration
Questions 151-180

151. The five personal values that describe the most effective and well-functioning teams include honesty, discipline, creativity, humility, and
    A. Curiosity.
    B. Personal accomplishments.
    C. Work-life balance.
    D. Certifications.

152. A nurse care coordinator is conducting a teaching session with a patient who was recently diagnosed with a lower-extremity blood clot. The patient has concerns about whether his over-the-counter herbal supplements will interact with his new anticoagulation profile. The nurse is uncertain of the answer and invites the clinical pharmacist to answer the patient's specific questions. This is an example of what principle of team-based health care?
    A. Shared goals.
    B. Clear roles.
    C. Mutual trust.
    D. Effective communication.

153. The nurse care coordinator holds monthly staff meetings and discusses safety and quality standards, reviews access-to-care metrics, and solicits feedback on previous performance-improvement projects. After the meetings, the nurse care coordinator posts the "meeting minutes" on a staff communication wall and emails them to all staff including those who were not in attendance. What principle of team-based health care is demonstrated by the nurse care coordinator's actions?
    A. Clear roles.
    B. Mutual trust.
    C. Effective communication.
    D. Measurable processes.

154. A primary care team, consisting of a family physician, clerk, nurse care coordinator, and scheduler, decides to reduce the number of complaints about the doctor running late in clinic. The team decides to implement a process that gives patients up-to-the-minute feedback about any clinic or provider delays. The team will reassess whether this improves overall customer satisfaction and agrees to track patient wait times to improve clinic performance immediately and over time. What principle of team-based health care is demonstrated?
    A. Clear roles.
    B. Mutual trust.
    C. Effective communication.
    D. Measurable processes and outcomes.

155. The nurse care coordinator, a soft-spoken nurse with a soothing voice and genuine smile, is called by one of her team members to calm an upset patient. She is frequently called upon to mediate difficult patient interactions and facilitate tense staffing discussions. When called upon to manage such episodes, the nurse care coordinator is demonstrating what type of leadership?
    A. Designated leadership.
    B. Situational leadership.
    C. Utilitarian leadership.
    D. Authoritative leadership.

156. Which of the following is an identified characteristic of a high-performing team?
    A. Setting clear expectations for each member to take advantage of division of labor.
    B. Withholding information from patients and team members until they are emotionally and intellectually ready.
    C. Establishing individual goals that reflect patient/caregiver priorities.
    D. Inviting local hospital representatives to attend staff meetings to openly discuss how each other's actions impact on adverse events related to transitions.

157. The nurse care coordinator is leading a morning staff huddle. Which comment **BEST** reflects the team communicates effectively?
    A. "You forgot to verify the patient's insurance coverage. The patient will not be able to get the equipment today that the provider prescribed since the patient's insurance was not verified."
    B. "Dr. Ker has a full clinic today so I will be auto-forwarding all incoming calls to voice mail. Patients can leave a message and I'll get back to them later this week."
    C. "It has been a few months since you have assisted Dr. Hall with a pelvic examination. Let's review the steps and needed supplies so the visit goes as smoothly as possible. What questions do you have before we begin?"
    D. "That nurse practitioner and I really do not work well together. Can I be reassigned to work with someone else?"

158. A nurse care coordinator and a licensed vocational/practical nurse are newly hired to an ambulatory procedures unit. During the course of their first week, the two nurses found themselves frustrated because they were doing each other's workload while some priority patient care tasks were left undone. Both nurses are irritated with each other and other team members can sense the conflict. Which team development process does this demonstrate?
    A. Norming.
    B. Performing.
    C. Forming.
    D. Storming.

159. A nurse care coordinator is a diligent and valued team member. During team meetings and huddles she rarely contributes, but several staff members "speak up for her" and share her ideas on process improvements. What is the **BEST** way to address this team member?
    A. Review the position description with the nurse care coordinator and remind her participation is a critical element for which she is evaluated during performance reviews.
    B. Encourage her co-workers to continue to "speak up" for her; praise them openly for their innovative ideas; and reward those co-workers with "Quality Recognition Awards."
    C. Establish an environment of psychological safety among team members to remove fear of being seen as ignorant, disruptive, or incompetent.
    D. Acknowledge to the nurse care coordinator that she is apparently shy and set up a recurring meeting with her after each staff meeting to solicit her feedback and suggestions.

160. The team, which has been in place for 6 months, was convened to create a process with a local laboratory and transportation service for interfacility transportation of patients for specimen collection and processing. The team reports that its objectives have been met: cost-effective processes are in place, and patients and staff are reporting successes from both facilities. The team requests to stay together for 4-6 more months to continue to refine processes. Which team development process **BEST** describes this team?
    A. Forming.
    B. Performing.
    C. Norming.
    D. Storming.

161. Which of the following nursing practices utilize a vast array of technologies such as phone, fax, email, Internet, and interactive video to deliver health services?
    A. Case management.
    B. Transitional nursing.
    C. Telehealth nursing.
    D. Medical-surgical nursing.

162. A mother of five school-aged children calls her primary care clinic and is connected to the nurse care coordinator. The mother is inquiring about migraine medications she has been using successfully for several years. In the background, the nurse care coordinator can hear a young child crying, the TV is very loud. The mother sounds like she has been crying. After ensuring safety, the nurse care coordinator assesses her current pain, formulates a diagnostic statement, reviews her pain management plan, instructs her about which medication to take for her pain level, and determines to call her back within an hour to evaluate effectiveness of the interventions. What principle is the nurse care coordinator's actions demonstrating?
    A. Application of the nursing process in telehealth triage.
    B. Proficiency in use of clinic-approved decision-support tools.
    C. Need for ongoing professional development.
    D. Practices within the guidelines set forth by HIPAA.

163. The nurse care coordinator is newly assigned to the centralized call center for a community-based family medicine clinic. On her first day, she comments to her nursing supervisor: "This job is going to be easy for me because all I have to do is ask a few questions and document the advice I give." The supervisor's response will be based on what principle of effective communication using telehealth technology?
    A. The nurse care coordinator must recognize that CCTM skills necessary for effective communication must be adapted when the nurse is not in the physical presence of the patient.
    B. Non-face-to-face communication is simpler because the RN cannot visualize the patient's problems and only needs to hear the voice.
    C. The nurse care coordinator interprets information to increase understanding.
    D. Telecommunication decreases the need for establishing rapport and empathy with the patient because the nurse care coordinator and patient cannot visually see each other.

164. The nurse care coordinator must be able use telecommunications technology appropriately, safely, and efficiently to meet patient needs. What is a principle of best practices to maintain safety and confidentiality?
    A. The nurse care coordinator confirms with whom she is interacting while on the phone by asking a family member to listen on the call.
    B. Instead of contacting the practice's information technology manager, the nurse care coordinator contacts a friend to troubleshoot connectivity issues.
    C. The nurse care coordinator uses only the certified systems designed for secure management of data and health information.
    D. The nurse care coordinator maintains an open door policy for communication while using telecommunication technology.

165. Valuing patient preferences and accepting personal responsibility for performance is an example of what intrinsic characteristic?
    A. Knowledge.
    B. Skill.
    C. Attitude.
    D. Integrity.

166. During morning huddle, the care team is discussing care needed and how it will be delivered to a patient with diabetes mellitus. The nurse care coordinator knows the most critical way to effectively determine what care will be delivered and the method for delivery is to demonstrate which principle of teamwork and collaboration?
    A. Conduct a pre-visit chart review to identify gaps in care.
    B. Build strong interprofessional teams.
    C. Understand the nursing care plan for diabetes mellitus.
    D. Negotiate patient services with the patient, family, and interprofessional team.

167. The director of nursing is introducing the Patient-Centered Medical Home (PCMH) model of care to the staff. How is a basic outcome of team-based care that helps guide and accelerate team-based care effectiveness measured?
    A. Per capita cost.
    B. Experience of care.
    C. Population health outcomes.
    D. Processes and outcomes

168. "Ensuring patients have opportunities to voice their opinions regarding care and services received and have issues reviewed and resolved, without fear of recrimination," is a measurement criteria for which standard in *Scope and Standards of Practice for Professional Ambulatory Care Nursing* (2010)?
    A. Standard 10: Collegiality.
    B. Standard 11: Collaboration.
    C. Standard 12: Ethics.
    D. Standard 14: Environment.

169. Which of the following provides stimulating new approaches to providing care?
    A. American Recovery and Reinvestment Act of 2009.
    B. Supplemental Appropriations and Rescissions Act of 1998.
    C. Uniform Interstate Family Support Act of 2001.
    D. Emergency Supplemental Appropriations Act of 1999.

170. Application of which of the following Ambulatory Care Nursing Standards (AAACN, 2010) ensures there is an effective match between nurse care coordination self-assessment and patient care needs?
    A. Application of Standard 10: Collegiality.
    B. Application of Standard 11: Collaboration.
    C. Application of Standard 12: Ethics.
    D. Application of Standard 14: Environment.

171. During a monthly team meeting, the nurse care coordinator appointed a unit nurse to lead and organize a designated care team, to establish clear goals, and facilitate open communication and teamwork among team members. Which answer **BEST** describes the nurse care coordinator's leadership style?
    A. Situational.
    B. Designated.
    C. Authoritarian.
    D. Transformational.

172. Which of the following is an evidence-based teamwork system aimed at optimizing patient outcomes through improving communication and teamwork skills among team members across the health care delivery system?
    A. Team STEPPS.
    B. Daily Goals Checklist.
    C. Team Check-up Tool.
    D. Morning Briefing.

173. The five principles of team-based health care include effective communication, clear roles, shared goals, mutual trust, and
    A. shared achievement.
    B. enhanced access to care.
    C. quality and safety
    D. measurable processes and outcomes.

174. The lead nurse is developing CCTM competencies for the nursing staff using the essential elements of telehealth. The essential elements of telehealth include professional practice and which of the following?
    A. Communication and health care standards.
    B. Effective communication, technology know-how, and ethical standards.
    C. Technology know-how, communication, and compliance standards.
    D. Technology know-how, communication, and education standards.

175. What is the **BEST** way to build and sustain a CCTM primary care team?
    A. Hire only BSN-prepared nurses to lead the teams.
    B. Introduce inclusion of teamwork in orientation and continuing education.
    C. Organize collaborative team meetings with specialty practices.
    D. Allow the most experienced health care provider to lead the team.

176. Which of the following is the last step when using the nursing process in telehealth triage?
    A. Collaboratively develop an individualized plan of care.
    B. Identify desired outcomes.
    C. Evaluate the effectiveness of triage intervention.
    D. Implement plan/intervention.

177. The nurse care coordinator is triaging a patient via telecommunication technology and is having a difficult time understanding the patient's needs because the patient does not speak fluent English. What is the **BEST** action for the nurse to take?
    A. Utilize an approved language line or interpreter.
    B. Use active listening to best understand the patient's needs.
    C. Ask another nurse to speak with the patient.
    D. Speak with the patient's family member instead.

178. The nurse care coordinator must be knowledgeable of which legal standard to ensure patient privacy?
    A. Scope and Standards of Practice for Professional Telehealth.
    B. American Nurses Association Code of Ethics (2001).
    C. Health Insurance Portability and Accountability Act (HIPAA).
    D. Occupational Safety and Health Administration (OSHA).

179. During a telehealth encounter, the patient and the nurse care coordinator agreed on how the plan of care would be implemented. Which of the following **BEST** describes the nurse care coordinator's future responsibility with this patient?
    A. Document the plan of care in the patient's record.
    B. Notify the specialist of the plan of care.
    C. Follow-up with the patient when indicated.
    D. Give the patient a copy of the plan of care.

180. What is identified as a challenge of utilizing telecommunications?
    A. Engaging in passive listening.
    B. Establishing a therapeutic relationship with the patient.
    C. Involving other members of the health care team.
    D. Timely documentation.

181. How does the domain of patient advocacy work towards system improvement to support patient-centered care?
    A. Assuring patients maintain control of patient encounters and treatment while the nurse care coordinator acts in a consultative role.
    B. Providing information about treatment options and plans, assessing patients' abilities, evaluating care and treatment, and communicating with other health care providers.
    C. Supporting and empowering patients to make informed decisions, navigate the health care system to access appropriate care and build strong partnerships with providers.
    D. Developing and updating organizational policies that define process and outcome indicators related to care coordination.

182. What is one example of how the nurse care coordinator as advocate in the CCTM Model utilizes behavior change science?
    A. Empowerment of patients to ensure control over their own care by helping the individual assume more of his or her own health-promoting activities.
    B. Assessment of patients' health literacy.
    C. Facilitating patient access to necessary and appropriate services while educating the patient, family, or caregiver regarding available resources through "teach-back" method.
    D. Motivational interviewing.

Questions 183 and 184 refer to the following patient case.

A patient with diabetes mellitus and middle-stage Alzheimer's disease experienced an acute care hospitalization due to a hypoglycemic episode. The patient was discharged home where the patient lives with a daughter who is the sole caregiver.

183. How does the nurse care coordinator **BEST** demonstrate the CCTM domain of advocacy?
    A. Calls patient within 48 hours of discharge, provides pharmacy information, monitors blood glucose by telehealth, facilitates PCP appointment, assesses daughter's knowledge of disease process, completes medication reconciliation, communicates patient status with PCP.
    B. Calls patient within 48 hours of discharge, schedules PCP appointment, instructs daughter to record the patient's blood glucose readings four times daily and bring the readings to the PCP appointment, and facilitates coordination of transportation.
    C. Calls the daughter within 48 hours of discharge to review the discharge instructions and confirm understanding follow-up needs; documenting the interaction in the EHR, including background, analysis of problems, and recommendations in preparation for PCP.
    D. Calls patient within 48-hours of discharge to review the discharge instructions; reassures the daughter as caregiver; informs the daughter of available resources, including those in the health care system, community, and those at local, and state levels.

184. During the post-discharge telephone call, the nurse care coordinator recognizes the patient's daughter sounds stressed and overwhelmed in her caregiver role. The daughter reports she is unable to work due to her mother's care needs, and is concerned with health care costs. The nurse care coordinator recognizes the need for support and assistance. When the nurse care coordinator performs a comprehensive assessment to identify actual and potential barriers to care, what else should the nurse care coordinator include with the assessment of finances, transportation, and health literacy?
    A. Lack of preventative care.
    B. Behavioral health.
    C. Psychosocial.
    D. Health disparities.

185. What action does the nurse care coordinator take to demonstrate commitment as a CCTM patient advocate to facilitate development and updating of organizational policies related to care coordination?
    A. Participating on Clinical Practice Committees (CPC).
    B. Becoming proficient in health care reform as described by the Patient Protection and Affordable Care Act (PPACA).
    C. Recognizing system barriers to patient access specific to underserved populations.
    D. Valuing active participation by nurses in federal policy formation.

186. The nurse care coordinator has established the knowledge, skills, and attitudes (KSA) for effective CCTM. What action demonstrates the ability to discuss principles of effective communication and the value of active partnerships with patients and surrogates in planning, implementation, and evaluation of care?
    A. Acting with strict honesty and integrity in relationships with patients, families, and team members.
    B. Communicating patient values, preferences, and expressed needs to other members of the health care team.
    C. Providing access to many resources across settings and providers.
    D. Participating in open dialogue and deliberation regarding ethical issues.

187. What is the **BEST** action for the nurse care coordinator to demonstrate being a key member of interprofessional coalitions as effective political strategists for influencing health policy?
    A. Engagement in partnerships with physicians, pharmacists, and other health care professionals to influence transformation on behalf of patients and families.
    B. Participation on patient safety and quality assurance committees.
    C. Advocating for National Database of Nursing Quality Indicators (NDNQI) outcome measures that reflect nurse care coordinator contributions to CCTM.
    D. Following the nursing professional code of ethics that states the nurse's primary commitment is to the patient.

188. The nurse care coordinator collaborates with a patient who has COPD and hypertension in setting an I-SMART goal during a telephone visit. The patient is a smoker, but feels it is more important to lose weight than to quit smoking. How does the nurse care coordinator demonstrate the domain of advocacy when supporting the choice for a goal to lose weight *rather* than the goal to quit smoking?
    A. Providing an opportunity for the patient to participate in planning care.
    B. Promoting the ethical principle of autonomy.
    C. Utilizing behavioral change science.
    D. Utilizing problem-solving skills and techniques to reconcile differing points of view between patient and providers.

189. When the nurse care coordinator develops a dietitian consult for the patient based on his educational needs for healthy weight loss; establishes patient agreement with the plan; practices nonjudgmental listening, planning, and evaluation of care; and involves other disciplines, the nurse care coordinator is displaying what core ethical principle of patient advocacy?
    A. Justice.
    B. Fidelity.
    C. Moral courage.
    D. Beneficence.

190. The nurse care coordinator recognizes the importance of customizing a plan of care consistent with the patient's values and needs. The nurse care coordinator applauds the choice for the health-promoting activity of losing weight. What principle of advocacy is the nurse care coordinator demonstrating?
    A. Providing access to resources across settings and providers.
    B. Communicating patient values, preferences, and expressed needs to other members of the health care team.
    C. Supporting the patient's right to self-determine a course of action and support independent decision-making.
    D. Valuing the patient's expertise with own health and symptoms.

191. The nurse care coordinator works in the ED. A patient who has a history of schizophrenia and homelessness, and frequent visits to the ED, presents with complaints of abdominal pain. Following care of the patient, the nurse care coordinator prepares the patient for discharge to include a referral to a social worker. The social worker contacts community resources to establish a site for shelter due to the patient's lack of housing. The nurse care coordinator demonstrates her knowledge of what fundamental understanding of the advocacy role in the care of underserved and vulnerable populations?
    A. Emergency departments and walk-in clinics are often the first choice for homeless, underserved, and frail elderly individuals requiring medical attention.
    B. The ethical principle of justice refers to protecting confidentiality and ethics an evidence-based framework.
    C. Customization of the plan of care needs to be consistent with meeting the patient's medical needs.
    D. The nursing assessment encompasses the total patient, including medical, behavioral, and socioeconomic.

192. A patient who is considered intellectually and developmentally disabled (I/DD), visits the ED frequently and lacks a primary care provider. The ED team coordinates the patient's care with a primary medical home. Why is the coordination with a primary medical home appropriate specifically for this patient?
    A. Many primary medical homes support the health care providers' desired outcomes of cost-effective adaptation and self-care.
    B. There are publically financed programs that support care needs and access to behavioral health and long-term services for patients with I/DD.
    C. Mary primary medical homes recognize system barriers to patient access, and know how to navigate these barriers.
    D. The primary medical home is the best option due to lack of care delivery models to address complex service needs of the I/DD population.

193. A patient without medical insurance was recently discharged from an inpatient stay for heart failure. This patient presents as a new patient for a follow-up visit at the primary care medical home clinic. The nurse care coordinator demonstrates knowledge of what fundamental understanding of the advocacy role in the care of underserved and vulnerable populations?
    A. The patient needs to recognize the signs and symptoms of exacerbation of heart failure and when to seek help.
    B. The association between health disparities and hospital readmissions.
    C. Publicly financed programs pay for many I/DD services.
    D. The duty to serve as a voice for the patient across settings and disciplines.

194. Which of the following demonstrates the nurse care coordinator's role as an advocate?
    A. Documenting using standardized or electronic tools to ensure portability of care.
    B. Assuring the patient views the nurse care coordinator as educator and problem solver.
    C. Assessing patient eagerness to solve problems, readiness to learn, and access to learning resources.
    D. Assessing for patient understanding and knowledge, and interest in sharing information with community.

195. In the policy development process in organizations with or seeking Magnet® designation, what must the organization **EXPLICITLY** identify?
    A. Building robust primary care models will mitigate the need for more expensive acute care services.
    B. Principles of change management are embraced universally.
    C. Nursing professional code of ethics states the nurse care coordinator's primary commitment is to the patient.
    D. Ambulatory nursing perspective is essential in describing care coordination activities.

196. The nurse care coordinator is on a hospital council at a hospital seeking Magnet® designation. What is the nurse care coordinator's **MOST** important contribution for Magnet® designation?
    A. Support evidence-based practice for best outcomes.
    B. Be aware of policy that impacts nursing practice and support compliance.
    C. Incorporate interprofessional collaboration when appropriate.
    D. Continue to advocate for NDNQI outcome measures.

197. The nurse care coordinator is seeking opportunities in public policy development and health care reform, and understands long-term solutions related to patient access must be built into public policy. To participate as an advocate, which of the following is an appropriate action for the nurse care coordinator?
    A. Engage in policy work through involvement in professional nursing organizations.
    B. Start a community-based grassroots effort to share intuitive concerns.
    C. Gather peers to discuss current health care issues in the hospital-based setting.
    D. Discuss politics while at work and start a home-based focus group.

198. The nurse care coordinator understands that moral courage is an essential skill for the role and is based on what principle of advocacy?
    A. Preserve integrity.
    B. Justify independent action.
    C. Support intuitive knowledge.
    D. Establish physician buy-in.

199. The nurse care coordinator understands the concept of keeping a commitment, based upon the virtue of caring. This demonstrates what ethical principle?
    A. Beneficence.
    B. Fidelity.
    C. Justice.
    D. Autonomy.

200. The nurse care coordinator is committed to improving CCTM and would like to become involved in advocacy at the policy level. What is the **BEST** team for this nurse care coordinator to become involved with?
    A. Community grassroots effort committed to blogging and use of social media to influence policy.
    B. A group of nurse care coordinators focused on policy that impacts pay for nurse care coordinators starting home care businesses with increased salaries.
    C. An interprofessional coalition aimed at influencing health policy, offering opportunity to become involved in state and national-level policy work.
    D. A group of nurse care coordinators aimed at identifying policies impacting credentialing and non-nursing caregiver groups.

Notes

1.	A	B	C	D
2.	A	B	C	D
3.	A	B	C	D
4.	A	B	C	D
5.	A	B	C	D
6.	A	B	C	D
7.	A	B	C	D
8.	A	B	C	D
9.	A	B	C	D
10.	A	B	C	D
11.	A	B	C	D
12.	A	B	C	D
13.	A	B	C	D
14.	A	B	C	D
15.	A	B	C	D
16.	A	B	C	D
17.	A	B	C	D
18.	A	B	C	D
19.	A	B	C	D
20.	A	B	C	D
21.	A	B	C	D
22.	A	B	C	D
23.	A	B	C	D
24.	A	B	C	D
25.	A	B	C	D
26.	A	B	C	D
27.	A	B	C	D
28.	A	B	C	D
29.	A	B	C	D
30.	A	B	C	D
31.	A	B	C	D
32.	A	B	C	D
33.	A	B	C	D
34.	A	B	C	D
35.	A	B	C	D
36.	A	B	C	D
37.	A	B	C	D
38.	A	B	C	D
39.	A	B	C	D
40.	A	B	C	D
41.	A	B	C	D
42.	A	B	C	D
43.	A	B	C	D
44.	A	B	C	D
45.	A	B	C	D
46.	A	B	C	D
47.	A	B	C	D
48.	A	B	C	D
49.	A	B	C	D
50.	A	B	C	D

51.	A	B	C	D
52.	A	B	C	D
53.	A	B	C	D
54.	A	B	C	D
55.	A	B	C	D
56.	A	B	C	D
57.	A	B	C	D
58.	A	B	C	D
59.	A	B	C	D
60.	A	B	C	D
61.	A	B	C	D
62.	A	B	C	D
63.	A	B	C	D
64.	A	B	C	D
65.	A	B	C	D
66.	A	B	C	D
67.	A	B	C	D
68.	A	B	C	D
69.	A	B	C	D
70.	A	B	C	D
71.	A	B	C	D
72.	A	B	C	D
73.	A	B	C	D
74.	A	B	C	D
75.	A	B	C	D
76.	A	B	C	D
77.	A	B	C	D
78.	A	B	C	D
79.	A	B	C	D
80.	A	B	C	D
81.	A	B	C	D
82.	A	B	C	D
83.	A	B	C	D
84.	A	B	C	D
85.	A	B	C	D
86.	A	B	C	D
87.	A	B	C	D
88.	A	B	C	D
89.	A	B	C	D
90.	A	B	C	D
91.	A	B	C	D
92.	A	B	C	D
93.	A	B	C	D
94.	A	B	C	D
95.	A	B	C	D
96.	A	B	C	D
97.	A	B	C	D
98.	A	B	C	D
99.	A	B	C	D
100.	A	B	C	D

101.	A	B	C	D		151.	A	B	C	D
102.	A	B	C	D		152.	A	B	C	D
103.	A	B	C	D		153.	A	B	C	D
104.	A	B	C	D		154.	A	B	C	D
105.	A	B	C	D		155.	A	B	C	D
106.	A	B	C	D		156.	A	B	C	D
107.	A	B	C	D		157.	A	B	C	D
108.	A	B	C	D		158.	A	B	C	D
109.	A	B	C	D		159.	A	B	C	D
110.	A	B	C	D		160.	A	B	C	D
111.	A	B	C	D		161.	A	B	C	D
112.	A	B	C	D		162.	A	B	C	D
113.	A	B	C	D		163.	A	B	C	D
114.	A	B	C	D		164.	A	B	C	D
115.	A	B	C	D		165.	A	B	C	D
116.	A	B	C	D		166.	A	B	C	D
117.	A	B	C	D		167.	A	B	C	D
118.	A	B	C	D		168.	A	B	C	D
119.	A	B	C	D		169.	A	B	C	D
120.	A	B	C	D		170.	A	B	C	D
121.	A	B	C	D		171.	A	B	C	D
122.	A	B	C	D		172.	A	B	C	D
123.	A	B	C	D		173.	A	B	C	D
124.	A	B	C	D		174.	A	B	C	D
125.	A	B	C	D		175.	A	B	C	D
126.	A	B	C	D		176.	A	B	C	D
127.	A	B	C	D		177.	A	B	C	D
128.	A	B	C	D		178.	A	B	C	D
129.	A	B	C	D		179.	A	B	C	D
130.	A	B	C	D		180.	A	B	C	D
131.	A	B	C	D		181.	A	B	C	D
132.	A	B	C	D		182.	A	B	C	D
133.	A	B	C	D		183.	A	B	C	D
134.	A	B	C	D		184.	A	B	C	D
135.	A	B	C	D		185.	A	B	C	D
136.	A	B	C	D		186.	A	B	C	D
137.	A	B	C	D		187.	A	B	C	D
138.	A	B	C	D		188.	A	B	C	D
139.	A	B	C	D		189.	A	B	C	D
140.	A	B	C	D		190.	A	B	C	D
141.	A	B	C	D		191.	A	B	C	D
142.	A	B	C	D		192.	A	B	C	D
143.	A	B	C	D		193.	A	B	C	D
144.	A	B	C	D		194.	A	B	C	D
145.	A	B	C	D		195.	A	B	C	D
146.	A	B	C	D		196.	A	B	C	D
147.	A	B	C	D		197.	A	B	C	D
148.	A	B	C	D		198.	A	B	C	D
149.	A	B	C	D		199.	A	B	C	D
150.	A	B	C	D		200.	A	B	C	D

Answer Key for
Care Coordination and Transition Management (CCTM) Review Questions

This answer key provides the correct answer for each question along with the rationale for why the answer is correct. The third column provides the reference page number in the *CCTM Core Curriculum* for each rationale.

CCTM Domain I: Communication and Transition Throughout the Care Continuum		Questions 1-14
Question Number	**Correct Answer**	***CCTM Core Curriculum* Page**
1.	A	103
Rationale: Access to transitional pieces of critical information contained in these documents facilitates a timely, efficient way to share information between providers and acute care sites.		
2.	C	103
Rationale: Issues with medication management are the most common cause of adverse events in transitional care.		
3.	B	103
Rationale: A shared electronic health record allows all team members to develop and share a plan of care and patient goals.		
4.	D	142-143
Rationale: Specialists, disease management clinics, and home care all need to be included in a common communication tool to provide a shared, coordinated plan of care and identify patient goals longitudinally.		
5.	C	145
Rationale: The BOOST tool identifies high-risk patients on admission and targets interventions with the 8Ps screening tool. Other models include Transitional Care Model (Naylor), Coleman's Care Transition Model, Project RED, and State Action on Avoidable Re-hospitalizations (STARR).		
6.	B	102
Rationale: Standardized tools such as SBAR or I-PASS increase the chances of a successful hand-off by applying consistent communication templates for information exchange in transitions of care.		
7.	A	111
Rationale: Information systems can be developed with safeguards and alerts based on evidence and available technology. Information systems are only one tool to safeguard protected health information. Information systems cannot guarantee patient understanding of the plan of care.		
8.	D	146
Rationale: Honoring active partnership with patients or their designated participants in planning, implementing, and evaluating care empowers them to become involved in the health care process. Goals for care can be longitudinal as well as specific for a care site.		
9.	D	154
Rationale: Lack of transportation for follow-up appointments is one barrier for patients which contributes to their inability to follow-up on the plan of care. Care coordinators can reduce that barrier by linking with community resources for transportation.		
10.	B	143
Rationale: Transitions from pediatric care to young adult is often overlooked as a transition of care. Changes in the patient's minority status may necessitate RN support in navigating the health system.		
11.	A	106
Rationale: Collaboration and open communication within teams are essential to achieve quality patient care during care transitions.		
12.	C	146
Rationale: Nurse care coordinators analyze patient centeredness of care in the context of patient past experience and educational/health literacy level. Cultural considerations need to be integrated into the plan of care.		
13.	A	146-147
Rationale: Nurse care coordinators help motivate patients to become involved in their care decisions and value their involvement. Activating patients for adherence and involvement in their treatment plans directly impacts health outcomes.		
14.	A	103
Rationale: Medication injuries are the most common adverse event reported related to communication failures during transitions of care.		

Answer Key for
Care Coordination and Transition Management (CCTM) Review Questions

CCTM Domain I: Communication and Transition Throughout the Care Continuum		Questions 15-26
Question Number	**Correct Answer**	**CCTM Core Curriculum Page**
15.	A	142
Rationale: Transitional care coordination between hospitals and primary care physicians is the most likely to reduce adverse events and readmission rates.		
16.	C	102
Rationale: Medically fragile and at-risk patients benefit from communication that is effective and thorough between all members of the care team, patients, and caregivers regardless of their setting.		
17.	C	103
Rationale: Lack of familiarity between patients and providers, such as hospitalists caring for patients in the in-patient setting but not outside of the hospital, can lead to lapses in communication and information transfer between patients and providers. The primary care team may be re-engaged through an office visit after discharge.		
18.	B	142
Rationale: The increased focus on quality of transitions is aimed at helping patients self-manage their illness at home and prevent after-hospital adverse events and readmissions.		
19.	C	154
Rationale: Health literacy impacts the patient's ability to understand or use information in ways that promote and maintain good health. "Teach-back" is a method used to validate a patient's understanding of the tool or skill provided for his or her health promotion.		
20.	B	101
Rationale: Ineffective communication is the most reported cause of sentinel events in U.S. hospitals (Dufault et al., 2010); 80% of mistakes happen because good communication failed or wasn't present at all. This also increases the likelihood of medication errors.		
21.	A	102
Rationale: Other elements are comprehensive assessment with goals and preferences, implementation of evidence-based plan of transitional care, care that is initiated at hospital admission and extends beyond discharge, engagement of patients and family, and coordinating services during and following the hospitalization. Having a mechanism to gather and share information is the key to all the other elements, for without good communication and information sharing, mistakes happen and care is not the best.		
22.	D	102
Rationale: The lack of hand-off communication is a huge risk, as there is possibly no information shared between care levels during transition. The other answers are all good forms of communication and, therefore, wouldn't be considered risk factors of inadequate communication.		
23.	B	103
Rationale: Hospital readmissions continue to be a risk of ineffective care transitions. If the patient doesn't have the proper follow-up, equipment, services, medication, and education, he or she will not be able to follow the plan of care properly.		
24.	B	107
Rationale: As seen with the PACT teams used at VA hospitals, team collaboration on transitions of care, care management, patient education, and communication are all the result of team building and collaboration, not only within the PACT teams themselves, but also throughout the community of care providers that the patient experiences. Continuity of care starts collaboration.		
25.	D	108
Rationale: The critical appraisal of research and evidence summaries would inform the nurse care coordinator of best practices for best outcomes, supporting a change in practice, such as patient education.		
26.	A	108
Rationale: Providing guidance on how to manage overlaps is a great strategy for leaders to use. Guidance allows for suggestions and feedback rather than dictating rules and policies that may not allow for flexibility.		

CCTM Domain I: Communication and Transition Throughout the Care Continuum		Questions 27-38
Question Number	**Correct Answer**	**CCTM Core Curriculum Page**
27.	B	104

Rationale: The Bridge Model utilizes master's-prepared social workers and includes three phases of intervention: pre-discharge, post-discharge, and follow-up. It was developed by Rush University Medical Center.

28.	A	105

Rationale: Sending the patient home with a reconciled, printed medication list ensures he or she has the most current medication information for self-administration of his or her medications, available refills, and dosage information. Ensuring the next appointment is scheduled makes certain the appointment is set for the appropriate clinically indicated time frame and allows the patient input as to his or her availability. This decreases the chance of missed opportunities.

29.	C	105

Rationale: Geriatric Resources for Assessment and Care of Elders. The NP and the social worker team together to develop care plans and meet the needs of low-income seniors, using GRACE-based protocols and a tracking system to monitor longitudinal progress.

30.	B	141

Rationale: By definition, transition of care is a range of time-specific services that complement primary care and ensure continuity of care between medical care settings.

31	D	146

Rationale: "Patient-centered care coordination is a core professional standard and competency for all registered nursing practice. ...the registered nurse is integral to patient care quality, satisfaction, and the effective and efficient use of health care resources. Registered nurses are qualified and educated for the role of care coordination, especially for high risk and vulnerable populations" (ANA, 2012, para 2).

32.	B	143

Rationale: Deficiencies in communication between health care providers within a setting or across settings influence transitions of care. The perception that responsibility for the patient ends at discharge might prevent important communication between care providers.

33.	C	143

Rationale: CCTP was designed to help those at risk for hospital readmission by providing in-depth coordination of transitions of care. BOOST is a care model of CCTP.

34.	A	148

Rationale: Good communication practices minimize the risk of hand-offs not being complete. Risks of poor communication include missing information, medication errors, and lack of patient education.

35.	A	154

Rationale: Follow-up phone calls and appointments are always appropriate after hospitalization to assess immediate needs and adherence to plan of care and for complications. Sending health literature can be done at any time and is not an element of a high-risk plan of support.

36.	A	154

Rationale: Patient support is the element of the assessment for risk of adverse events post-discharge that can be addressed with a phone call by the health care team to ensure adherence to the plan of care, assess immediate needs, and assess for complications.

37.	C	154

Rationale: A follow-up phone call can address issues of poor health literacy to assess adherence to the plan of care and complications. The patient can be evaluated for the ability to do "teach-back" and for symptoms he or she may not otherwise be able to recognize.

38.	B	142

Rationale: Information must be communicated to the acute care setting on current prescription and over-the counter medication use.

Answer Key for
Care Coordination and Transition Management (CCTM) Review Questions

CCTM Domain I: Communication and Transition Throughout the Care Continuum		Questions 39-40
Question Number	Correct Answer	CCTM Core Curriculum Page
39.	B	155

Rationale: Initiation of palliative care should not be started until the patient and/or family has discussed prognosis with the care team and agreed to palliative care. During this conversation, benefits and services related to palliative care can be discussed. Once agreed upon, goals and therapeutic options can be discussed as well as bothersome symptoms the patient/family may wish to have specifically managed.

40.	B	104

Rationale: The nurse care coordinator can educate patients on self-management decision-making tools, such as what to do with insulin dosing if they are sick; this promotes activation for self-care.

CCTM Domain II: Education, Engagement, Coaching, and Counseling of Patients, Caregivers, and Support Network		Questions 41-50
41.	A	24

Rationale: By asking the patient to talk about his previous experience with IV infusion therapy, the nurse care coordinator honors the patient's experience. This patient has had previous experience with IV infusion therapy and will identify what he needs to know.

42.	D	26

Rationale: Asking questions that require more than a yes/no answer encourages the patient to discuss his health concerns.

43.	B	27

Rationale: Asking the patient to validate his understanding by using his own words or "teach-back" validates the patient's understanding.

44.	D	24

Rationale: Cognitive therapy identifies the need for the learner to gain attention, receive information, and identify how that information is used. Learners need to process information to demonstrate understanding. Multiple sessions may be required, but are not part of the theory.

45.	A	26

Rationale: Avoid communicating with the use of idioms. Examples of idioms are "heads up" or "feeling blue."

46.	B	25

Rationale: Look at the patient not the interpreter is a fundamental practice principle supporting the use of interpreters to utilize knowledge of culture to work toward a positive health outcome (DHHS, 2001).

47.	D	26

Rationale: Use collective knowledge of the health care team to assess, plan, implement, and evaluate information shared and alter plans as needs change by coordinating the health care team to target the same health literacy level and education.

48.	A	28

Rationale: Knowledge of team roles help the patient to know how different members can address different needs. Partnering with the team helps patients identify and monitor treatment and self-care goals as well as include providers in discussion of values and preferences about decisions.

49.	A	28

Rationale: Competency for patient-centered planning includes understanding and seeking the values and preferences of the patient/family/community regarding health and illness as well as being flexible in problem solving with a commitment to the patient and family.

50.	A	23

Rationale: Patient education is the process of influencing patient behavior and producing the changes in knowledge, attitudes, and skills necessary to maintain or improve health.

Answer Key for
Care Coordination and Transition Management (CCTM) Review Questions

CCTM Domain II: Education, Engagement, Coaching, and Counseling of Patients, Caregivers, and Support Network		Questions 51-63
Question Number	Correct Answer	*CCTM Core Curriculum* Page
51.	A	27-28

Rationale: Evaluating reliability in health information includes looking for authorship/sponsorship of material. Sources of reliable material include government, institutions of higher education, non-profit and for-profit organizations. Additional elements to consider when evaluating reliability include information based on evidence or research, date of the material, as well as updates.

| 52. | A | 28 |

Rationale: Five core self-management skills include problem-solving, decision-making, utilization of resources, partnerships with health care providers, and taking action to achieve health goals.

| 53. | A | 32 |

Rationale: The competency elements include defining information, communication, and education; assessing patient and family readiness; and creating an environment of communication and questioning that empowers the patient/family to engage in planning care.

| 54. | C | 25 |

Rationale: Break content into smaller, understandable "chunks" of information to increase patient understanding.

| 55. | A | 29 |

Rationale: Attitudes for patient-centered planning include but are not limited to seeing health care situations through the patient's eyes, being flexible and seeking to solve problems with a commitment to the patient and family, and respecting and encouraging expression of patient values, preferences, and expressed needs.

| 56. | A | 34 |

Rationale: Acknowledge the tension that may exist between patient rights and the organizational responsibility for professional and ethical care.

| 57. | D | 26 |

Rationale: "Ask Me 3" questions include: What is my main problem? What do I need to do? and Why is it important for me to do this?

| 58. | B | 27-28 |

Rationale: The date of when the publication was published provides information on whether the information is current or outdated. There is more reliability of information that is based on evidence or research and authored through a professional organization or government agency.

| 59. | B | 163 |

Rationale: Mobile technology and Cloud computing play a major role in CCTM. As nurse care coordinators advise and educate patients, it is important to assess the Internet sources of education using criteria to ensure the information is a valid and reliable source of evidence-based content.

| 60. | C | 163 |

Rationale: Nursing informatics is defined by the American Nurses Association (2010) as a "specialty that integrates nursing science, computer science, and information science to manage and communicate data, information, knowledge, and wisdom in nursing practice."

| 61. | C | 164 |

Rationale: Health information technology (HIT) can support the activities related to care coordination, facilitate transfer of information, enable communication between parties in different locations, and provide real-time decision support.

| 62. | A | 164 |

Rationale: The ability to navigate the EHR demonstrates the nurse care coordinator's ability to locate information to support care coordination activities.

| 63. | A | 164 |

Rationale: This response is most supportive for the RN-CCTM Model as the nurse care coordinator can be proactive in identifying the patient's need. This is an example of how HIT can support functions related to CCTM.

Answer Key for
Care Coordination and Transition Management (CCTM) Review Questions

CCTM Domain II: Education, Engagement, Coaching, and Counseling of Patients, Caregivers, and Support Network		Questions 64-76
Question Number	**Correct Answer**	***CCTM Core Curriculum* Page**
64.	A	165

Rationale: The nurse care coordinator can be proactive and plan patient education with the information stated on the report. This is an example of how HIT can support functions related to CCTM.

65.	A	165

Rationale: The use of clinical decision-support tools in CCTM requires the recognition that they are to be utilized to support decision-making in concert with critical thinking and clinical judgment rather than dictate practice.

66.	D	165

Rationale: Information and technology are utilized to communicate, manage knowledge, mitigate error, and support decision-making.

67.	D	166

Rationale: HIT supports team collaboration and can be designed to provide alerts when pertinent (e.g., medication) information is missing when the patient transitions from one setting to another.

68.	A	166

Rationale: An example of how a decision-support system might operate in a clinical setting is the scheduling of immunizations. The system would ask for input of the child's date of birth, weight, immunization history, and other pertinent facts. The algorithm in the inference engine would be used to provide a recommendation for the next immunization to be scheduled.

69.	B	167

Rationale: The term *syndromic surveillance* applies to surveillance using health-related data (typically symptom clusters) that precede a given diagnosis and signal a sufficient probability of a number of cases or a potential population outbreak that would warrant further response.

70.	D	167

Rationale: The element is for reports that inform the team and front-line workers of progress and problem areas to address.

71.	C	38

Rationale: If patient-centered goals and participation are valued as team outcomes, then the nurse will be able to communicate the patient's values, preferences, and expressed needs to other members of the health care team.

72.	C	38-39

Rationale: The Registered Nurse in Care Coordination and Transition Management (RN in CCTM) is the day-to-day communicator in an outpatient setting and therefore can strive to include the patient and family in the team. In-person care coordinator-only visits as well as telephone and email communication can facilitate this interaction effectively.

73.	C	42-43

Rationale: Advising provides information about health risks and benefits of change. Evidence-based guidelines are also shared with patients to encourage participation.

74.	A	38

Rationale: Pre-contemplation is the time when the individual is not aware of a need to change behavior.

75.	D	40

Rationale: Goals are set collaboratively. Make SMART goals: Specific, Measurable, Attainable, Realistic, Timely.

76.	A	168

Rationale: Use of the National Quality Strategy focuses on care coordination by aligning efforts of the use of HIT to focus on effective communication to coordinate care.

Answer Key for
Care Coordination and Transition Management (CCTM) Review Questions

CCTM Domain II: Education, Engagement, Coaching, and Counseling of Patients, Caregivers, and Support Network		Questions 77-80
Question Number	Correct Answer	CCTM Core Curriculum Page
77.	A	168

Rationale: Care coordination is the integration of care across the continuum of the patient's health care conditions, needs, and experiences that incorporates transfer of information.

78.	A	168

Rationale: Primary care providers are the pivotal members of the health care team. Care coordination depends on the EHR to facilitate communication and transfer of information. Share information within and outside practice, integrate specialty care, and transfer info across all settings of care.

79.	A	168

Rationale: The Act fosters adoption of "meaningful use" of certified EHRs to improve quality and reduce health costs.

80.	C	168

Rationale: Both systems are dependent on the EHR to facilitate communication and transfer of information.

CCTM Domain III: Population and Health Management		Questions 81-88
81.	A	113

Rationale: "Keeping a population as healthy as possible" describes the foundation/focus of population health.

82.	C	113

Rationale: Describes how organizations organize themselves to address population health; the nurse care coordinator will need to have an understanding of population health organizational structure.

83.	B	115

Rationale: The Population Health Management Model identifies the steps in the process beginning with population identification, continues with enrollment and engagement, delivery modalities, patient-centered interventions, and ends with evaluations. The framework is useful to organize the work that needs to occur in population health.

84.	D	115

Rationale: Wagner's Chronic Care Model was developed to improve chronic illness care, a significant part of population health. Several elements are identified that support the patient-provider interactions and can result in improved outcomes.

85.	C	116

Rationale: The population health version of the assessment portion of the nursing process: The more data you are able to obtain the more accurate your plan of care.

86.	A	116

Rationale: "Patients 50 years old and over needing colorectal screening" is the best response to demonstrate the principle of population identification. To manage population health effectively, an organization must be able to track and monitor the health of individual patients. The use of population management tools are an efficient resource (e.g., registries, analytic tools) to track and monitor select population characteristics.

87.	B	117

Rationale: "Stratify patients in the practice by risk of getting sick or sicker" is the best response as it addresses the goal of PHM. "Stratify patients in the practice by disease diagnosis" as noted on this page was the traditional way to stratify patients, but if the individual with the disease is well controlled, involved in care, and manages his or her disease, this patient should not be included in an initial stratification if the nurse care coordinator is looking at those most likely to become sick or sicker.

88.	D	118

Rationale: A cornerstone of PHM is the ability to be proactive in closing gaps in care. A registry provides the CCTM nurse with information related to potential gaps in care. Transitions in care across the continuum require closing gaps in care.

Answer Key for
Care Coordination and Transition Management (CCTM) Review Questions

CCTM Domain III: Population and Health Management		Questions 89-100
Question Number	**Correct Answer**	***CCTM Core Curriculum* Page**
89.	C	119

Rationale: Team-based interventions require staff and resources that are beyond what the primary care physicians can provide; to include planning and implementing care groups, working with patients outside of the office visit, and monitoring effectiveness.

90.	A	120

Rationale: Attending or leading daily huddles to discuss needed patient interventions is included to document the importance of team communication.

91.	C	123 & 124

Rationale: Nursing informatics through the implementation of EHRs provides knowledge to manage and communicate data and review information.

92.	A	123 & 124

Rationale: Registries are a fundamental tool used by the nurse care coordinator to prioritize patients with high-risk clinical conditions, serious unmet clinical need for outreach, and intervention to manage outcomes.

93.	B	123 &124

Rationale: Registries are critical tools used to identify gaps in care such as lack of post-discharge follow-up after hospitalization missed preventative screening and unfilled prescriptions.

94.	C	121

Rationale: Telephone outreach can be part of the framework a nurse care coordinator implements for patient engagement. It is identified that patients demonstrate better outcomes when they self-manage symptoms, engage in activities that maintain function and reduce health decline, are involved in treatment and diagnostic choices, and collaborate with providers.

95.	C	117-118

Rationale: Project BOOST's 8Ps Risk Assessment Tool identifies patient factors linked to high rates of adverse events after discharge. The tool is completed on admission, identifying patients at risk for adverse events post-hospitalization. The P – "principle diagnosis" – is an area assessed, and COPD is listed as high risk.

96.	A	79

Rationale: Data, both objective and subjective, contribute to accurate transition management assessment.

97.	A	121 & 122

Rationale: PAM stands for "Patient Activation Measure," a valid scale demonstrating patient's level of engagement/potential to collaborate with the health care team.

98.	B	122

Rationale: There is a growing body of evidence that demonstrates patients who are engaged in their care are more likely to be adherent to the plan of care and achieve better outcomes. One component of patient engagement is the knowledge patients with low PAM and high disease burden may require RN and physician-level resources for patient engagement.

99.	D	79, 116, & 117

Rationale: The initial nurse care coordinator task is to collect evidence-based data to determine the population's needs; in a healthy population, the focus is on prevention of conditions that are evidenced in the population served.

100.	A	117

Rationale: "Practices that have a population with a higher stratification of healthy people focus their care efforts on prevention and wellness." The CDC lists each vaccine in the "A" option for the age group as a recommendation; the CDC also recommends HPV for both men and women.

Answer Key for
Care Coordination and Transition Management (CCTM) Review Questions

CCTM Domain III: Population and Health Management		Questions 101-112
Question Number	**Correct Answer**	*CCTM Core Curriculum* **Page**
101.	C	116
Rationale: Health plan eligibility and administrative data are the most comprehensive data for building a registry, which must cover the entire population.		
102.	D	117, 122, & 124
Rationale: Care management stratification focuses on whether patients are ill enough to require ongoing support from a care manager, utilizing clinical outcome measures (number of seizures), health care utilization measures (ED visits), and quality-of-life measures (missed days from work or school).		
103.	A	118
Rationale: Identification of gaps in care is an essential component of the nurse care coordinator and PHM impacting program outcomes.		
104.	C	120
Rationale: There is a growing body of evidence that demonstrates patients who are more engaged in their care are more likely to be adherent to the plan of care and achieve better outcomes. (Hibbard, Greene, & Overton, 2013)		
105.	B	118
Rationale: Evidence-based clinical outcomes measures for chronic conditions are the foundation for registries, which highlight potential gaps and provide structure for individualized care plans.		
106.	B	123
Rationale: Care coordination EHR documentation tools utilize automated outreach and reminders to ensure patients are reminded to receive preventative screenings and routine exams to promote wellness and support optimal disease management.		
107.	A	123
Rationale: Automated systems based on the EHR population registry capture the entire eligible population and are not person-dependent.		
108.	D	123
Rationale: Developing a patient registry in the EHR enables teams to record and share information across systems to facilitate accurate and timely access to patient information. Developing a database with limited access or documenting in a generic location in the EHR will not promote communication or care effectively among the health care team.		
109.	B	124
Rationale: Decision-support tools involve clinical alerts to the nurse care coordinator to highlight the need for preventative health support, nursing intervention, and/or change in risk stratification.		
110.	C	125
Rationale: Measurement of the impact of population health across different strata is required to assure equitable care across significant strata, such as racial or socioeconomic groups.		
111.	C	124
Rationale: PHM tools are built on evidence-based and measureable outcomes related to the population: clinical outcome measures (A1c results), health care utilization measures (readmissions), and quality of life (QOL) measures (missed days from work or school). Billing and electronic communication are not directly related to QOL measures.		
112.	A	116
Rationale: Organizations store multiple sources of data in a data warehouse; clinical data may come from the EHR, billing, and claims.		

Answer Key for
Care Coordination and Transition Management (CCTM) Review Questions

CCTM Domain III: Population and Health Management		Questions 113-120
Question Number	**Correct Answer**	***CCTM Core Curriculum* Page**
113.	B	125

Rationale: HITECH addresses EHR utilization, privacy, and security concerns through several provisions that strengthen enforcement of the HIPAA rules.

114.	D	116

Rationale: HIEs allow for the storage and sharing of information across payers, practice settings, and tracking systems.

115.	C	123 & 125

Rationale: Informatics integrates computer and information science to manage and communicate data, information, knowledge, and wisdom. Informatics is the structure into which evidence-based practice is infused, to promote safety and identify gaps which are addressed via quality improvement processes.

116.	B	125

Rationale: Quality improvement practice has the aim of optimizing safety, utilizing evidence-based practice to establish goals, and the tools within the realm of informatics to manage the data and identify gaps.

117.	B	127

Rationale: Compliance is active involvement in one's care; patient-centered care involves analyzing the reasons for barriers to active involvement/compliance to care.

118.	D	128

Rationale: Health literacy is influenced by education level, educational and cultural experiences, and social and educational backgrounds.

119.	B	133

Rationale: Clinical practice guidelines are developed from clinical research and evidence-based best practices for a given disease or condition with the goal of optimizing care with wise stewardship of health care resources.

120.	A	134

Rationale: Quality improvement involves acknowledging the importance of population-relevant benchmarks from comprehensive databases as a tool to measure/estimate the quality of care in a given PHM system.

CCTM Domain IV: Patient-Centered Care Planning and Support for Self-Management		Questions 121-124
121.	C	47

Rationale: The Psychosocial Assessment Tool is a Patient Health Questionnaire with 2 or 9 questions (PHQ-2 or 9) that assesses patients for signs and symptoms of depression. It is a screening tool used as a first-step approach (Kroenke, Spitzer, & Williams, 2003).

122.	A	48

Rationale: Ms. Frank applies the use of knowledge of the Modified Caregiver Strain Index: "Caregivers may be prone to depression, grief, fatigue, financial hardship, and changes in social relationships. It is a useful screening tool to identify families who would benefit from a more comprehensive assessment of the care giving experience by identifying appropriate interventions needed to help the caregiver" (Onega, 2013, p. 1).

123.	D	49

Rationale: The patient's medical record or electronic health record is a useful tool in the early phase of patient assessment. Questions to be posed include:
a. When was the patient last seen by his or primary care provider?
b. Has he or she missed several appointments?
c. Are medications up to date (expired or need refill)?
d. Are the patient's recommended preventive care guidelines up to date?

124.	D	49

Rationale: Based upon practice guidelines for age, gender, and diagnoses, the nurse can identify needed tests and screenings, such a foot exam, referral for retinal exam, and an A1c for a patient with diabeties.

CCTM Domain IV: Patient-Centered Care Planning and Support for Self-Management		Questions 125-138
Question Number	**Correct Answer**	***CCTM Core Curriculum* Page**
125.	A	49

Rationale: It is necessary to plan for the patient's visit in advance so outstanding test results, recommended preventive care, and PCP orders are obtained before the visit. This includes a review of missing labs, x-rays, and specialty referrals (e.g., retinal exam), and immunizations with PCP.

126.	A	50

Rationale: Key – A strategy to proactively identify and outreach to at-risk patients to develop patient-centered care planning is to use chronic disease-based models, such as diabetes-specific models.

127.	B	50

Rationale: Patient engagement – once the patient is identified as high risk, next step is to contact the patient and/or caregiver for intake and assessment. Explain you are available to help with transportation, medications, disease-specific questions, and to coordinate care overall.

128.	C	51

Rationale: Listen for "change talk." One of the first steps in helping patients make the argument for change is being able to recognize change talk (Rollnick et al., 2008).

129.	D	51

Rationale: Motivational interviewing is a patient-centered counseling style for addressing the common problem of ambivalence about change by paying particular attention to the language of change.

130.	B	51

Rationale: Building rapport involves engaging the patient and supporting him in a nonjudgmental manner. Open-ended questions facilitate patient engagement.

131.	C	52

Rationale: Goal setting – based on assessment, discuss goals that are agreeable to the patient and/or caregiver. The care plan is patient driven and goals are patient, not provider centered.

132.	B	53

Rationale: Education – once the goals have been determined, the patient and nurse care coordinator in CCTM agree on a specified date and time for follow-up. The patient leaves with culturally specific, literacy-based education material to review.

133.	A	54

Rationale: "The term evidence-based practice is used to describe activities or treatments that are based on results of clinical research, not hunches or suspicions" (Tabloski, 2009, p. 53).

134.	C	55

Rationale: Quality measures are tracked utilizing the Healthcare Effectiveness Data and Information Set (HEDIS™), a tool used by more than 90% of America's health plans to measure performance on important dimensions of care and service.

135.	B	55

Rationale: A common "red flag" when monitoring a patient's progress includes hospital readmissions including all-cause 30-day readmissions, because it indicates the patient is not able to fully self-manage when discharged.

136.	B	51

Rationale: One of the barriers to patient engagement is low health literacy (education), because the patient may not comprehend the education and may be self-conscious about his or her limited ability.

137.	C	49

Rationale: The Patient Activation Measure assessment gauges the knowledge, skills, and confidence essential to manage one's own health and health care.

138.	D	51

Rationale: Motivational interviewing is characterized as evocative.

Answer Key for
Care Coordination and Transition Management (CCTM) Review Questions

CCTM Domain IV: Patient-Centered Care Planning and Support for Self-Management		Questions 139-150
Question Number	**Correct Answer**	***CCTM Core Curriculum* Page**
139.	C	66

Rationale: The first step is to assess her knowledge and her current practices, then reinforce and build upon this foundation of knowledge and health behaviors.

140.	D	66

Rationale: The nurse needs to understand what perceptions Ms. Miller has about lifestyle changes and self-management efforts Ms. Miller has tried and dismissed as unhelpful.

141.	C	69

Rationale: The goals must be the goals of the patient, not those of the health care team. The nurse care coordinator can begin exploring with the patient about her goal, using a tool such as the I-SMART acronym.

142.	B	69

Rationale: Self-efficacy is enhanced by success in solving one's own problems.

143.	A	67-68

Rationale: Self-management barriers may be physical, psychological, cognitive, economic, or social and cultural. One cannot assume that it is lack of an effective medical plan or lack of money. Smoking cessation is important, but may not have an immediate impact on his ED utilization.

144.	C	70-71

Rationale: Motivational interviewing uses communication techniques such as open-ended questions, affirmation, and reflection. It is effective in some, but not all patient populations. Option B describes the peer coaching method and D describes the "Five A's" approach.

145.	C	68

Rationale: Sedating medications may affect cognition and the patient's ability to self-manage.

146.	C	69

Rationale: Economic barriers may impact many aspects of Ms. Miller's self-management of her health. One needs to understand her perception and priorities to collaboratively develop goals and a plan for her to execute.

147.	B	70

Rationale: Self-evaluation and tailoring requires the patient to measure success against individualized goals. Ms. Frank appears to have a plan and is evaluating her success and adjusting actions.

148.	A	69

Rationale: The contemplative stage of readiness to change is described by Fava, Velicer, and Prochaska (1995) as that time in which the person is considering the change within 6 months.

149.	C	69

Rationale: Reflective thinking by a patient or family is described as considering their readiness and ability to change, the barrier to the change, and their personal beliefs.

150.	C	71

Rationale: Battersby et al. (2010) report that value of follow-up is enhanced when it is specific to the patient's data, monitoring progress toward goals and problem-solving for that patient's specific barriers. Follow-up includes appointments, case-management via telephone, tele-monitoring, and personalized reminders, but there is not one method that is best in all situations. Follow-up is effective for both self-management of chronic conditions and risk factor reduction.

Answer Key for
Care Coordination and Transition Management (CCTM) Review Questions

CCTM Domain V: Teamwork and Interprofessional Collaboration		Questions 151-163
Question Number	**Correct Answer**	***CCTM Core Curriculum* Page**
151.	A	90
Rationale: The five personal values identifying and characterizing the most effective members of well-functioning teams include honesty, discipline, creativity, humility, and curiosity.		
152.	B	90
Rationale: There are clear expectations for each team member's functions, responsibilities, and accountabilities, which optimize the team's efficiency and often make it possible for the team to take advantage of division of labor. The nurse acknowledges uncertainty of drug-herbal interactions; therefore, correctly refers the patient to the clinical pharmacist.		
153.	C	90
Rationale: The team prioritizes and continuously refines its communication skills. It has consistent channels for candid and complete communication, which are accessed and used by all team members across all settings.		
154.	D	90
Rationale: The team agrees on and implements reliable and timely feedback on successes and failures in both the functioning of the team and achievement of the team's goals. These are used to track and improve performance immediately and over time.		
155.	B	92
Rationale: Situational leaders can be any team member who has the skills to manage a situation at hand; and they may act as facilitator when teams are not functioning well.		
156.	A	92
Rationale: High-functioning teams work to establish clear expectations for each member to take advantage of all human resources and divide labor.		
157.	C	92-93
Rationale: Huddles are an effective method for communicating. Reflection includes use of explicit observations, questions, and discussions of processes and outcomes.		
158.	D	93
Rationale: Storming occurs when members are establishing their position within the team, which can cause conflict and the need for clarification.		
159.	C	94
Rationale: Strong team leadership involves removing barriers that hinder idea sharing.		
160.	B	93
Rationale: A performing team shares the vision, team members identify areas for continued refinement, and goals are achieved.		
161.	C	175
Rationale: The competency definition of telehealth is "the inclusive term used to describe the wide range of health services delivered, managed, and coordinated by all health related disciplines via electronic information and telecommunications technologies" (Greenberg, Espensen, Becker, & Cartwright, 2003, p. 8).		
162.	A	176
Rationale: Telehealth triage requires nurses to perform assessments, formulate diagnostic statements related to the nature of the problem, identify desired outcomes, collaborate with patients on plan of care, and evaluate the effectiveness of triage recommendations.		
163.	A	177
Rationale: The RN in CCTM must identify and implement communication strategies that accurately and effectively elicit and provide information to patients, nurses, and other team members. Depending on the telecommunication technology used, the nurse will be communicating via visual, auditory, or written means or a combination of these. Therefore, the RN in CCTM must recognize the skills necessary for effective communication must be adapted when the nurse is not in the physical presence of the patient, his or her family/caregiver, or other members of the health care team (Rutenberg & Greenberg, 2012).		

CCTM Domain V: Teamwork and Interprofessional Collaboration		Questions 164-176
Question Number	**Correct Answer**	***CCTM Core Curriculum* Page**
164.	C	177

Rationale: The nurse care coordinator maintains patient safety and confidentiality when using telehealth technology by using certified practices and systems for secure management of data and health information.

165.	C	187

Rationale: Values are intrinsic characteristics. This is an example of an attitude.

166.	B	89

Rationale: Care is given not just to the patient, but also to caregivers and families. The IOM says professionals need to use skills that build relationships with patients and their peers. The most critical way in which CCTM will be carried out effectively is through the building of strong interprofessional teams.

167.	D	90

Rationale: The team agrees on and implements reliable and timely feedback on successes and failures in both the functioning of the team and achievement of the team's goals. These are used to track and improve performance immediately and over time.

168.	C	91

Rationale: The discussion of the scope of practice for professional ambulatory care nursing included ethics as one of the main characteristics. It is further defined by ten components; to include patients having opportunities to voice their opinions.

169.	A	90

Rationale: The American Recovery and Reinvestment Act of 2009 and the Patient Protection and Affordable Care Act of 2010 are cited as stimulating new approaches to providing care. A common element of these new approaches, of which the Medical Home Model is just one example, is that they depend on interprofessional teamwork and on team-based care.

170.	D	91

Rationale: The scope of practice for professional ambulatory care nursing includes environment as one of the main characteristics. It is further defined by three components, one of which addresses the requirement to match patient care needs with nurse self-assessment to ensure safety (AAACN, 2010).

171.	B	92

Rationale: Designated leaders are persons assigned to lead and organize a designated care team, establish clear goals, and facilitate open communication and teamwork among team members.

172.	A	91

Rationale: Team STEPPS was developed by the U.S. Department of Defense's Patient Safety Program in collaboration with the Agency for Healthcare Research and Quality. The evidence upon which Team STEPPS is based demonstrates effective teamwork and collaboration result in improved patient safety, fewer errors, improved patient outcomes, improved process outcomes, improved patient satisfaction, and improved satisfaction among team members.

173.	D	90

Rationale: The five principles of team-based care are effective communication, clear roles, shared goals, mutual trust, and measurable processes and outcomes.

174.	B	176

Rationale: Professional practice, effective communication, technology know-how, and ethical standards are the essential elements of telehealth.

175.	B	11

Rationale: Per the Logic Model of the CCTM, teamwork and continuing education are activities that lend to a more engaged/less silo-ish health care team.

176.	C	176

Rationale: Evaluating the effectiveness of triage interventions demonstrates the final step in the nursing process.

Answer Key for
Care Coordination and Transition Management (CCTM) Review Questions

CCTM Domain V: Teamwork and Interprofessional Collaboration		Questions 177-180
Question Number	**Correct Answer**	***CCTM Core Curriculum* Page**
177.	A	177
Rationale: When necessary, the nurse care coordinator needs to recognize the need and enlist the services of an interpreter for language interpretation.		
178.	C	176
Rationale: The Health Insurance Portability and Accountability Act (HIPAA) is the legal standard, which ensures secure electronic access and privacy regulations for health data.		
179.	C	180
Rationale: The nurse care coordinator must recognize the telehealth encounter does not end with implementation of the plan of care. The nurse has a responsibility to follow-up, when indicated, to measure attainment of desired outcomes and assure patient safety.		
180.	D	177
Rationale: Clear and prompt documentation of telehealth interactions needs to occur to ensure current information and plans of care are accessible to members of the health care team.		
CCTM Domain VI: Advocacy		Questions 181-188
181.	C	13
Rationale: Patient advocacy is the support and empowerment of patients to make informed decisions, navigate the health care system to access appropriate care, and build strong partnerships with providers, while working toward system improvement to support patient-centered care.		
182.	D	15
Rationale: Motivational interviewing is an effective behavioral change tool where patients are guided towards talking about change in their own words. Through motivational interviewing, the nurse care coordinator as advocate moves patients to optimal levels of health based on their current situation.		
183.	A	15
Rationale: A best plan of care addresses all the elements important in CCTM advocacy. Acting as patient advocate, the nurse care coordinator in CCTM provides information about treatment options and plans, assesses the patient's (caregiver) abilities, evaluates care and treatment, and communicates with other health care providers.		
184.	C	15
Rationale: When negotiating services with the daughter, the goal is to move the mother as patient to an optimal level of health based on her current situation. The nurse care coordinator as advocate in the CCTM Model completes a comprehensive assessment to identify actual or potential barriers that include financial, transportation, psychosocial, and health literacy.		
185.	A	7
Rationale: Membership on a health system, hospital, service line, or department CPC provides opportunities for nurse care coordinators to introduce or contribute to nursing policies related to CCTM.		
186.	B	19
Rationale: The ability to communicate patient values, preferences, and expressed needs to other members of the health care team is the necessary skill for effective communication when partnering with patients and/or surrogates for patient planning, implementation, and evaluation needs.		
187.	A	18
Rationale: As the most trusted professionals in health care, nurses have a potentially powerful voice. Interprofessional coalitions are effective political strategies for influencing health policy and should include nurse care coordinators.		
188.	B	15
Rationale: By helping patients assume responsibility of their own health-promoting activities and goals, nurse care coordinators practice ethically by promoting patient autonomy. Autonomy is the right to self-determine a course of action and support of patients' independent decision-making.		

Answer Key for
Care Coordination and Transition Management (CCTM) Review Questions

CCTM Domain VI: Advocacy		Questions 189-200
Question Number	**Correct Answer**	***CCTM Core Curriculum* Page**
189.	D	15

Rationale: Beneficence is defined as nonjudgmental listening, planning, and evaluation of care as well as involvement of other disciplines and understanding the patient's vulnerability.

190.	C	15

Rationale: The ethical principle of autonomy is defined as supporting the patient's right to self-determine a course of action and support independent decision-making. Autonomy is a component of the philosophical framework for the nurse care coordinator to examine values as they relate to human behaviors.

191.	A	17

Rationale: Knowing emergency departments and walk-in clinics are often the first choice for homeless, underserved, and frail elderly individuals requiring medical attention, practicing advocacy requires the RN in CCTM to assist in navigating the patient to the appropriate level of care and service.

192.	B	17

Rationale: A patient who meets the criteria for publicly financed programs based on his intellectual and developmental disability. Referring this patient to a Medical Home that supports need for care and access to behavioral health and long-term services is appropriate for the role of the nurse care coordinator in the role as advocate for the care of the underserved and vulnerable population.

193.	B	17

Rationale: "The association between health disparities and hospital readmissions" addresses the role of advocacy in the care of underserved and vulnerable populations. The patient needs to be identified with the factors associated with vulnerable populations.

194.	A	15

Rationale: Moral courage is an essential skill for nurses as advocates. Ensuring portability of care by documenting using standardized or electronic tools is identified in the *CCTM Core Curriculum* as an essential element of advocacy for the nurse care coordinator. The documentation method described supports optimal care coordination and transition management needs of the patient and family.

195.	D	17

Rationale: Ambulatory nursing perspective is essential in describing care coordination activities contributing to nursing excellence in an organization seeking Magnet designation.

196.	D	17

Rationale: The role of advocacy in organizational policy development states the ambulatory nurse must continue to advocate for National Database of Nursing Quality Indicators outcome measures, which reflect ambulatory nurse contributions to care coordination and transition management.

197.	A	18

Rationale: Policy development and health care reform require care coordination and transition management activities by ambulatory nurses are reflected in public policy. Work through involvement in professional nursing organizations at the state and national levels is identified in the role of advocacy for the nurse care coordinator.

198.	A	15

Rationale: Moral courage is identified by four elements: ability to overcome fear and stand up for core values and ethical obligations; knowledge of professional ethical obligations; required in individual and in organizational advocacy; and preservation of integrity as "an aspect of wholeness of character" in nursing's professional code of ethics.

199.	B	15

Rationale: The ethical principle of fidelity is defined by the concept of keeping commitment based on the virtue of caring.

200.	C	18

Rationale: To achieve concrete system-wide change, nurse care coordinators must engage in broad partnerships to influence transformation on behalf of patients and families. Engaging in coalition partnerships offer a collective voice and can influence positive change.

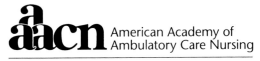 American Academy of
Ambulatory Care Nursing

Many settings. Multiple roles. One unifying specialty.

Mission

Advance the art and science of ambulatory care nursing.

Vision

Professional registered nurses are the recognized leaders in ambulatory care environments. They are valued and rewarded as essential to quality health care.

Strategic Message

AAACN is a welcoming, unifying community for registered nurses in all ambulatory care settings. This professional organization offers:
- Connections with others in similar roles.
- Help in advancing practice and leadership skills.
- Advocacy that promotes greater appreciation for the specialty of ambulatory care nursing.

Core Values

Individually and collectively, our members are guided by our deep belief in:
- Responsible health care delivery for individuals, families, and communities.
- Visionary and accountable leadership.
- Productive partnerships, alliances, and collaborations.
- Appreciation of diversity.
- Continual advancement of professional ambulatory care nursing practice.

Goals

1. *Serve Our Members* – Enhance the professional growth and career advancement of our members.
2. *Expand Our Influence* – Expand the influence of AAACN and ambulatory care nurses to achieve a greater positive impact on the quality of ambulatory care.
3. *Strengthen Our Core* – Ensure a healthy organization committed to serving our members and expanding our influence.

Initiatives

Initiative 1 – Care Coordination and Transition Management (CCTM)
Initiative 2 – Ambulatory Nurse Sensitive Indicators
Initiative 3 – RN Residency Program
Initiative 4 – Telehealth Nursing Practice

Membership

Over 3,000 registered nurses who practice in varying ambulatory care settings such as hospital-based outpatient clinics/centers, solo/group medical practices, telehealth call centers, university hospitals, community hospitals, military and VA settings, managed care/HMOs/PPOs, colleges/educational institutions, patient homes, and freestanding facilities. Members are managers and supervisors, administrators and directors, staff nurses, care coordinators, educators, consultants, advanced practice nurses, and researchers.

Membership Benefits

Academy membership benefits include discounted rates to the AAACN National Preconference and Conference offering multiple practice innovations, industry exhibits, and numerous networking opportunities. Other benefits include distance learning programs, special member rates on publications and the fee to take the ANCC ambulatory care nursing certification exam or the MSNCB Care Coordination and Transition Management exam; the bimonthly newsletter - *ViewPoint;* subscription to **one** of three bimonthly journals – *Nursing Economic$, MEDSURG Nursing, or Pediatric Nursing*; opportunity to join a special interest group in the area of: Leadership, Patient/Staff Education, Pediatrics, Telehealth Nursing Practice, Veterans Affairs, and Tri-Service Military; awards and scholarship programs; access to national experts and colleagues through AAACN's online membership directory, monthly E-newsletter, community discussions, online library, an Expert Panel, web site **aaacn.org**; and online Career Center.

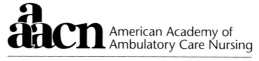

American Academy of
Ambulatory Care Nursing

Many settings. Multiple roles. One unifying specialty.

AAACN Publications/Education Resources

▶ *Scope and Standards of Practice for Professional Ambulatory Care Nursing, 2010*

▶ *Core Curriculum for Ambulatory Care Nursing, 2013*

▶ *Ambulatory Care Nursing Certification Review Course Syllabus, 2015*

▶ *Ambulatory Care Nursing Orientation and Competency Assessment Guide, 2010*

▶ *Ambulatory Care Nursing Review Questions, 2013*

▶ *Care Coordination and Transition Management Core Curriculum Text, 2014*

▶ *Care Coordination and Transition Management Review Questions, 2016*

▶ *Scope and Standards of Practice for Registered Nurses in Care Coordination and Transition Management, 2015*

▶ *Scope and Standards of Practice for Professional Telehealth Nursing, 2011*

▶ *Telehealth Nursing Practice Essentials Textbook, Second Printing 2012*

AAACN Courses

▶ Care Coordination and Transition Management (CCTM) Courses, 2015, 2016

  • (www.aaacn.org/library or http://aaacn.org/cctm2

▶ Ambulatory Care Nursing Certification Review Course *(DVD and online), 2015*

▶ Ambulatory Care Nursing Certification Review Focused CE Series through Nurse.com

Position Statements/Paper

▶ *Nurse Licensure Compact (NLC) Position Statement*

▶ *The Role of the Registered Nurse in Ambulatory Care Position Statement*

▶ *The Role of the Registered Nurse in Ambulatory Care Position Paper*

Annual Conference

AAACN provides cutting-edge information and education at its annual conference, usually held in the month of March or April. Nurses from across the country as well as international colleagues come together to network, learn from each other, and share knowledge and skills. Renowned speakers in the field of ambulatory care present topics of current interest offering over 24 contact hours. An Exhibit Hall featuring the products and services of vendors serving the ambulatory care and telehealth community provides information and resources to attendees.

Certifications

AAACN values the importance of certification and promotes achieving this level of competency through its educational products to prepare nurses to take the ambulatory care nursing certification examination (www.nursecredentialing.org) AAACN strongly encourages all telehealth nurses to become certified in ambulatory care nursing. Because telehealth nurses provide nursing care to patients who are in ambulatory settings, they must possess the knowledge and competencies to provide ambulatory care appropriately. Ambulatory certification is and will continue to be the gold standard credential for any nursing position within ambulatory care.

AAACN collaborated with the Medical-Surgical Nursing Certification Board (MSNCB) to develop a certification exam in care coordination and transition management www.msncb.org/cctm. The exam is administered by the Center for Nursing Education and Testing (C-NET) at http://www.cnetnurse.com.

For More Information, Contact:

American Academy of Ambulatory Care Nursing
P.O. Box 56, Pitman, NJ 08071-0056
Phone: 800-262-6877
Fax: 856-589-7463
Email: aaacn@aaacn.com
Web site: www.aaacn.org

Notes

Care Coordination *and* **Transition Management** – *REVIEW QUESTIONS*

Notes

Notes